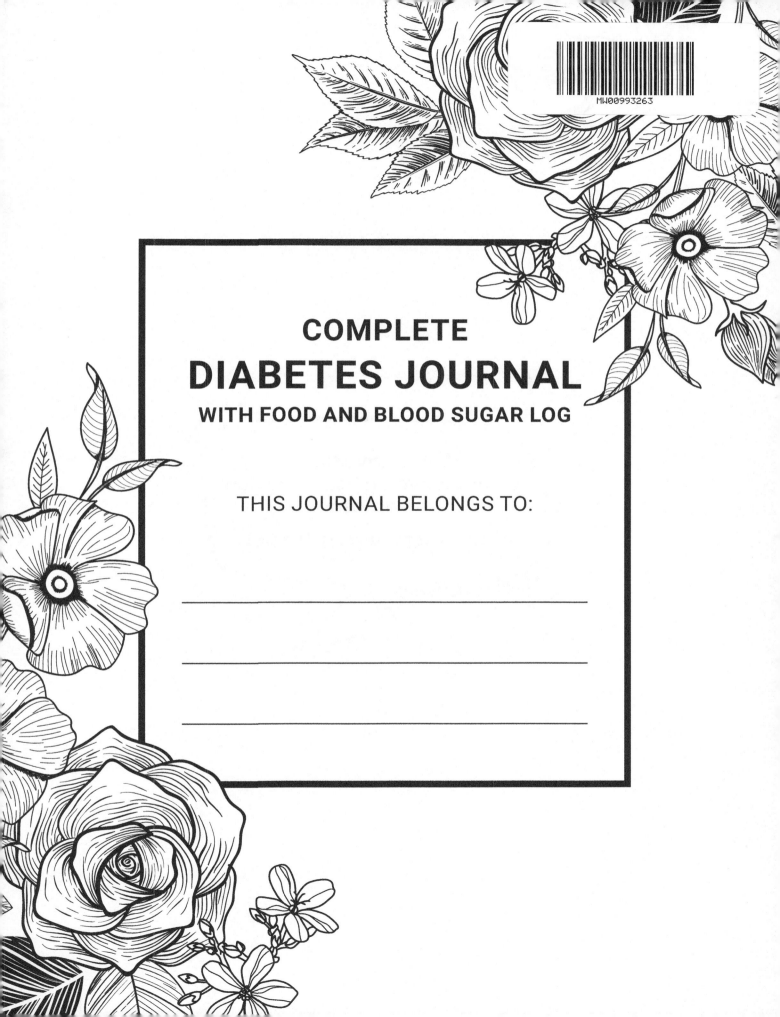

COMPLETE
DIABETES JOURNAL
WITH FOOD AND BLOOD SUGAR LOG

THIS JOURNAL BELONGS TO:

_____

_____

_____

If you have time,
please leave an honest review
on amazon.

It means the world to us!

Personal Information and Medical Contacts

Personal Information

Name:

Gender:

Date of Birth:

Blood Group:

Emergency Contact

Name:

Phone No:

Relationship:

Address:

Doctor Information

Name:

Phone No:

Notes:

Pharmacy Information

Name:

Phone No:

Notes:

Additional Notes

_____

_____

_____

_____

_____

_____

_____

_____

_____

Blood Sugar Reference Charts

Fasting Blood Sugar/Plasma Glucose(FBS/FPG)

Normal	less than 100 mg/dl
Pre-Diabetes	101 mg/dl to 125 mg/dl
Diabetes	126 mg/dl or higher

A1C / HBA1C

Normal	less than 5.7%
Pre-Diabetes	5.7% to 6.4%
Diabetes	6.5% or higher

Random Blood Sugar(RBS)

Normal	less than 200 mg/dl
Pre-Diabetes	N/A
Diabetes	200 mg/dl or higher

Doctor Appointments

Date: **Time:**

Place:

Doctor:

Reason:

Notes:

Next Visit:

Date: **Time:**

Place:

Doctor:

Reason:

Notes:

Next Visit:

Date: **Time:**

Place:

Doctor:

Reason:

Notes:

Next Visit:

Date: **Time:**

Place:

Doctor:

Reason:

Notes:

Next Visit:

Doctor Appointments

Date: Time:

Place:

Doctor:

Reason:

Notes:

Next Visit:

Date: Time:

Place:

Doctor:

Reason:

Notes:

Next Visit:

Date: Time:

Place:

Doctor:

Reason:

Notes:

Next Visit:

Date: Time:

Place:

Doctor:

Reason:

Notes:

Next Visit:

Medication Organizer

Date	Medication/Insulin/Supplement	Dosage/Description

Medication Organizer

Date	Medication/Insulin/Supplement	Dosage/Description

Tests,Labs & Checkups

F B S Target: _____	
Date	**Value**

A 1 C Target: _____	
Date	**Value**

B M I Target: _____	
Date	**Value**

Date	Test	Values	Notes

DATE: _____ SU | MO | TU | WE | TH | FR | SA   **Month/Week:** _____

FOOD, NUTRITION & MEDS

	Carbs	Sugar	Fiber	Protein	Fat	Calories
BREAKFAST Time: _____ Meds/Insulin: _____						
Breakfast Total						
SNACK 1 Time: _____ Meds/Insulin: _____						
Snack 1 Total						
LUNCH Time: _____ Meds/Insulin: _____						
Lunch Total						
SNACK 2 Time: _____ Meds/Insulin: _____						
Snack 2 Total						
DINNER Time: _____ Meds/Insulin: _____						
Dinner Total						
Total Nutrition for the Day						

Water Consumption ▢ ▢ ▢ ▢ ▢ ▢ ▢ ▢ ▢   _____

EXERCISE & ACTIVITY LOG

	Time/Duration	Intensity/Calories

BLOOD SUGAR LOG

	Blood Sugar Level	
	Before	**After**
WAKING UP Time: _____	Sleep Hrs: _____ Fast. Hrs: _____	
BREAKFAST		
SNACK 1		
LUNCH		
SNACK 2		
DINNER		
BEDTIME	Go to Sleep Time: _____	

BLOOD PRESSURE & WEIGHT

Time	SYS/DIA	Pulse

WEIGHT: _____

NOTES/SCHEDULE

7 am	
8 am	
9 am	
10 am	
11 am	
12 am	
1 pm	
2 pm	
3 pm	
4 pm	
5 pm	
6 pm	
7 pm	
8 pm	

DATE: _____ SU | MO | TU | WE | TH | FR | SA   **Month/Week:** _____

FOOD, NUTRITION & MEDS

	Carbs	Sugar	Fiber	Protein	Fat	Calories
BREAKFAST Time: _____ Meds/Insulin: _____						
Breakfast Total						
SNACK 1 Time: _____ Meds/Insulin: _____						
Snack 1 Total						
LUNCH Time: _____ Meds/Insulin: _____						
Lunch Total						
SNACK 2 Time: _____ Meds/Insulin: _____						
Snack 2 Total						
DINNER Time: _____ Meds/Insulin: _____						
Dinner Total						
Total Nutrition for the Day						

Water Consumption ▯ ▯ ▯ ▯ ▯ ▯ ▯ ▯ ▯ ▯ _____

EXERCISE & ACTIVITY LOG

	Time/Duration	Intensity/Calories

BLOOD SUGAR LOG

	Blood Sugar Level	
	Before	**After**
WAKING UP Time: _____	Sleep Hrs: _____ Fast. Hrs: _____	
BREAKFAST		
SNACK 1		
LUNCH		
SNACK 2		
DINNER		
BEDTIME	Go to Sleep Time: _____	

BLOOD PRESSURE & WEIGHT

Time	SYS/DIA	Pulse
WEIGHT: _____		

NOTES/SCHEDULE

7 am	
8 am	
9 am	
10 am	
11 am	
12 am	
1 pm	
2 pm	
3 pm	
4 pm	
5 pm	
6 pm	
7 pm	
8 pm	

DATE: _____   SU | MO | TU | WE | TH | FR | SA   **Month/Week:** _____

FOOD, NUTRITION & MEDS

	Carbs	Sugar	Fiber	Protein	Fat	Calories
BREAKFAST Time: _____ Meds/Insulin: _____						
Breakfast Total						
SNACK 1 Time: _____ Meds/Insulin: _____						
Snack 1 Total						
LUNCH Time: _____ Meds/Insulin: _____						
Lunch Total						
SNACK 2 Time: _____ Meds/Insulin: _____						
Snack 2 Total						
DINNER Time: _____ Meds/Insulin: _____						
Dinner Total						
Total Nutrition for the Day						

Water Consumption ▯ ▯ ▯ ▯ ▯ ▯ ▯ ▯ ▯ ▯ _____

EXERCISE & ACTIVITY LOG

	Time/Duration	Intensity/Calories

BLOOD SUGAR LOG

	Blood Sugar Level	
	Before	**After**
WAKING UP Time: _____	Sleep Hrs: _____ Fast. Hrs: _____	
BREAKFAST		
SNACK 1		
LUNCH		
SNACK 2		
DINNER		
BEDTIME	Go to Sleep Time: _____	

BLOOD PRESSURE & WEIGHT

Time	SYS/DIA	Pulse

WEIGHT: _____

NOTES/SCHEDULE

7 am	
8 am	
9 am	
10 am	
11 am	
12 am	
1 pm	
2 pm	
3 pm	
4 pm	
5 pm	
6 pm	
7 pm	
8 pm	

DATE: _____ SU | MO | TU | WE | TH | FR | SA   **Month/Week:** _____

FOOD, NUTRITION & MEDS

	Carbs	Sugar	Fiber	Protein	Fat	Calories
BREAKFAST Time: _____ Meds/Insulin: _____						
Breakfast Total						
SNACK 1 Time: _____ Meds/Insulin: _____						
Snack 1 Total						
LUNCH Time: _____ Meds/Insulin: _____						
Lunch Total						
SNACK 2 Time: _____ Meds/Insulin: _____						
Snack 2 Total						
DINNER Time: _____ Meds/Insulin: _____						
Dinner Total						
Total Nutrition for the Day						

Water Consumption ⬚ ⬚ ⬚ ⬚ ⬚ ⬚ ⬚ ⬚ ⬚ _____

EXERCISE & ACTIVITY LOG

	Time/Duration	Intensity/Calories

BLOOD SUGAR LOG

	Blood Sugar Level	
	Before	**After**
WAKING UP Time: _____	Sleep Hrs: _____ Fast. Hrs: _____	
BREAKFAST		
SNACK 1		
LUNCH		
SNACK 2		
DINNER		
BEDTIME	Go to Sleep Time: _____	

BLOOD PRESSURE & WEIGHT

Time	SYS/DIA	Pulse
WEIGHT: _____		

NOTES/SCHEDULE

7 am	
8 am	
9 am	
10 am	
11 am	
12 am	
1 pm	
2 pm	
3 pm	
4 pm	
5 pm	
6 pm	
7 pm	
8 pm	

DATE: _____ SU | MO | TU | WE | TH | FR | SA   **Month/Week:** _____

FOOD, NUTRITION & MEDS

		Carbs	Sugar	Fiber	Protein	Fat	Calories
BREAKFAST Time: _____	Meds/Insulin: _____						
	Breakfast Total						
SNACK 1 Time: _____	Meds/Insulin: _____						
	Snack 1 Total						
LUNCH Time: _____	Meds/Insulin: _____						
	Lunch Total						
SNACK 2 Time: _____	Meds/Insulin: _____						
	Snack 2 Total						
DINNER Time: _____	Meds/Insulin: _____						
	Dinner Total						
	Total Nutrition for the Day						

Water Consumption ☐ ☐ ☐ ☐ ☐ ☐ ☐ ☐ ☐ ☐   _____

EXERCISE & ACTIVITY LOG

	Time/Duration	Intensity/Calories

BLOOD SUGAR LOG

	Blood Sugar Level	
	Before	**After**
WAKING UP Time: _____	Sleep Hrs: _____ Fast. Hrs: _____	
BREAKFAST		
SNACK 1		
LUNCH		
SNACK 2		
DINNER		
BEDTIME	Go to Sleep Time: _____	

BLOOD PRESSURE & WEIGHT

Time	SYS/DIA	Pulse

WEIGHT: _____

NOTES/SCHEDULE

7 am	
8 am	
9 am	
10 am	
11 am	
12 am	
1 pm	
2 pm	
3 pm	
4 pm	
5 pm	
6 pm	
7 pm	
8 pm	

DATE: _____ SU | MO | TU | WE | TH | FR | SA   **Month/Week:** _____

FOOD, NUTRITION & MEDS

	Carbs	Sugar	Fiber	Protein	Fat	Calories

BREAKFAST Time: _____ Meds/Insulin: _____

	Carbs	Sugar	Fiber	Protein	Fat	Calories
Breakfast Total						

SNACK 1 Time: _____ Meds/Insulin: _____

	Carbs	Sugar	Fiber	Protein	Fat	Calories
Snack 1 Total						

LUNCH Time: _____ Meds/Insulin: _____

	Carbs	Sugar	Fiber	Protein	Fat	Calories
Lunch Total						

SNACK 2 Time: _____ Meds/Insulin: _____

	Carbs	Sugar	Fiber	Protein	Fat	Calories
Snack 2 Total						

DINNER Time: _____ Meds/Insulin: _____

	Carbs	Sugar	Fiber	Protein	Fat	Calories
Dinner Total						
Total Nutrition for the Day						

Water Consumption 🥛🥛🥛🥛🥛🥛🥛🥛🥛 _____

EXERCISE & ACTIVITY LOG

	Time/Duration	Intensity/Calories

BLOOD SUGAR LOG

	Blood Sugar Level	
	Before	**After**
WAKING UP Time: _____	Sleep Hrs: _____ Fast. Hrs: _____	
BREAKFAST		
SNACK 1		
LUNCH		
SNACK 2		
DINNER		
BEDTIME	Go to Sleep Time: _____	

BLOOD PRESSURE & WEIGHT

Time	SYS/DIA	Pulse
WEIGHT: _____		

NOTES/SCHEDULE

7 am	
8 am	
9 am	
10 am	
11 am	
12 am	
1 pm	
2 pm	
3 pm	
4 pm	
5 pm	
6 pm	
7 pm	
8 pm	

DATE: _____ SU | MO | TU | WE | TH | FR | SA **Month/Week:** _____

FOOD, NUTRITION & MEDS

	Carbs	Sugar	Fiber	Protein	Fat	Calories
BREAKFAST Time: _____ Meds/Insulin: _____						
Breakfast Total						
SNACK 1 Time: _____ Meds/Insulin: _____						
Snack 1 Total						
LUNCH Time: _____ Meds/Insulin: _____						
Lunch Total						
SNACK 2 Time: _____ Meds/Insulin: _____						
Snack 2 Total						
DINNER Time: _____ Meds/Insulin: _____						
Dinner Total						
Total Nutrition for the Day						

Water Consumption ☐ ☐ ☐ ☐ ☐ ☐ ☐ ☐ ☐ _____

BLOOD SUGAR LOG

	Blood Sugar Level	
	Before	**After**
WAKING UP Time: _____	Sleep Hrs: _____ Fast. Hrs: _____	
BREAKFAST		
SNACK 1		
LUNCH		
SNACK 2		
DINNER		
BEDTIME	Go to Sleep Time: _____	

BLOOD PRESSURE & WEIGHT

Time	SYS/DIA	Pulse
WEIGHT: _____		

NOTES/SCHEDULE

7 am	
8 am	
9 am	
10 am	
11 am	
12 am	
1 pm	
2 pm	
3 pm	
4 pm	
5 pm	
6 pm	
7 pm	
8 pm	

EXERCISE & ACTIVITY LOG

	Time/Duration	Intensity/Calories

DATE: _____ SU | MO | TU | WE | TH | FR | SA **Month/Week:** _____

FOOD, NUTRITION & MEDS

	Carbs	Sugar	Fiber	Protein	Fat	Calories
BREAKFAST Time: _____ Meds/Insulin: _____						
Breakfast Total						
SNACK 1 Time: _____ Meds/Insulin: _____						
Snack 1 Total						
LUNCH Time: _____ Meds/Insulin: _____						
Lunch Total						
SNACK 2 Time: _____ Meds/Insulin: _____						
Snack 2 Total						
DINNER Time: _____ Meds/Insulin: _____						
Dinner Total						
Total Nutrition for the Day						

Water Consumption ⬜ ⬜ ⬜ ⬜ ⬜ ⬜ ⬜ ⬜ ⬜ _____

EXERCISE & ACTIVITY LOG

	Time/Duration	Intensity/Calories

BLOOD SUGAR LOG

	Blood Sugar Level	
	Before	After
WAKING UP Time: _____	Sleep Hrs: _____ Fast. Hrs: _____	
BREAKFAST		
SNACK 1		
LUNCH		
SNACK 2		
DINNER		
BEDTIME	Go to Sleep Time: _____	

BLOOD PRESSURE & WEIGHT

Time	SYS/DIA	Pulse
WEIGHT: _____		

NOTES/SCHEDULE

7 am	
8 am	
9 am	
10 am	
11 am	
12 am	
1 pm	
2 pm	
3 pm	
4 pm	
5 pm	
6 pm	
7 pm	
8 pm	

DATE: _____   SU | MO | TU | WE | TH | FR | SA   **Month/Week:** _____

FOOD, NUTRITION & MEDS

	Carbs	Sugar	Fiber	Protein	Fat	Calories

BREAKFAST   Time: _____   Meds/Insulin: _____

Breakfast Total						

SNACK 1   Time: _____   Meds/Insulin: _____

Snack 1 Total						

LUNCH   Time: _____   Meds/Insulin: _____

Lunch Total						

SNACK 2   Time: _____   Meds/Insulin: _____

Snack 2 Total						

DINNER   Time: _____   Meds/Insulin: _____

Dinner Total						
Total Nutrition for the Day						

Water Consumption ▢ ▢ ▢ ▢ ▢ ▢ ▢ ▢ ▢ ▢   _____

EXERCISE & ACTIVITY LOG

	Time/Duration	Intensity/Calories

BLOOD SUGAR LOG

	Blood Sugar Level	
	Before	**After**
WAKING UP Time: _____	Sleep Hrs: _____ Fast. Hrs: _____	
BREAKFAST		
SNACK 1		
LUNCH		
SNACK 2		
DINNER		
BEDTIME	Go to Sleep Time: _____	

BLOOD PRESSURE & WEIGHT

Time	SYS/DIA	Pulse
WEIGHT: _____		

NOTES/SCHEDULE

7 am	
8 am	
9 am	
10 am	
11 am	
12 am	
1 pm	
2 pm	
3 pm	
4 pm	
5 pm	
6 pm	
7 pm	
8 pm	

DATE: _____   SU | MO | TU | WE | TH | FR | SA   **Month/Week:** _____

FOOD, NUTRITION & MEDS

	Carbs	Sugar	Fiber	Protein	Fat	Calories
BREAKFAST Time: _____ Meds/Insulin: _____						
Breakfast Total						
SNACK 1 Time: _____ Meds/Insulin: _____						
Snack 1 Total						
LUNCH Time: _____ Meds/Insulin: _____						
Lunch Total						
SNACK 2 Time: _____ Meds/Insulin: _____						
Snack 2 Total						
DINNER Time: _____ Meds/Insulin: _____						
Dinner Total						
Total Nutrition for the Day						

Water Consumption ▢ ▢ ▢ ▢ ▢ ▢ ▢ ▢ ▢ _____

EXERCISE & ACTIVITY LOG

	Time/Duration	Intensity/Calories

BLOOD SUGAR LOG

	Blood Sugar Level	
	Before	**After**
WAKING UP Time: _____	Sleep Hrs: _____ Fast. Hrs: _____	
BREAKFAST		
SNACK 1		
LUNCH		
SNACK 2		
DINNER		
BEDTIME	Go to Sleep Time: _____	

BLOOD PRESSURE & WEIGHT

Time	SYS/DIA	Pulse
WEIGHT: _____		

NOTES/SCHEDULE

7 am	
8 am	
9 am	
10 am	
11 am	
12 am	
1 pm	
2 pm	
3 pm	
4 pm	
5 pm	
6 pm	
7 pm	
8 pm	

DATE: _____ SU | MO | TU | WE | TH | FR | SA   **Month/Week:** _____

FOOD, NUTRITION & MEDS

	Carbs	Sugar	Fiber	Protein	Fat	Calories
BREAKFAST Time: _____ Meds/Insulin: _____						
Breakfast Total						
SNACK 1 Time: _____ Meds/Insulin: _____						
Snack 1 Total						
LUNCH Time: _____ Meds/Insulin: _____						
Lunch Total						
SNACK 2 Time: _____ Meds/Insulin: _____						
Snack 2 Total						
DINNER Time: _____ Meds/Insulin: _____						
Dinner Total						
Total Nutrition for the Day						

Water Consumption ⬜⬜⬜⬜⬜⬜⬜⬜⬜⬜ _____

BLOOD SUGAR LOG

	Blood Sugar Level	
	Before	**After**
WAKING UP Time: _____	Sleep Hrs: _____ Fast. Hrs: _____	
BREAKFAST		
SNACK 1		
LUNCH		
SNACK 2		
DINNER		
BEDTIME	Go to Sleep Time: _____	

BLOOD PRESSURE & WEIGHT

Time	SYS/DIA	Pulse
WEIGHT: _____		

NOTES/SCHEDULE

7 am	
8 am	
9 am	
10 am	
11 am	
12 am	
1 pm	
2 pm	
3 pm	
4 pm	
5 pm	
6 pm	
7 pm	
8 pm	

EXERCISE & ACTIVITY LOG

	Time/Duration	Intensity/Calories

DATE: _____ SU | MO | TU | WE | TH | FR | SA

Month/Week: _____

FOOD, NUTRITION & MEDS

	Carbs	Sugar	Fiber	Protein	Fat	Calories
BREAKFAST Time: _____ Meds/Insulin: _____						
Breakfast Total						
SNACK 1 Time: _____ Meds/Insulin: _____						
Snack 1 Total						
LUNCH Time: _____ Meds/Insulin: _____						
Lunch Total						
SNACK 2 Time: _____ Meds/Insulin: _____						
Snack 2 Total						
DINNER Time: _____ Meds/Insulin: _____						
Dinner Total						
Total Nutrition for the Day						

Water Consumption 🥛🥛🥛🥛🥛🥛🥛🥛🥛🥛 _____

BLOOD SUGAR LOG

	Blood Sugar Level	
	Before	After
WAKING UP Time: _____	Sleep Hrs: _____ Fast. Hrs: _____	
BREAKFAST		
SNACK 1		
LUNCH		
SNACK 2		
DINNER		
BEDTIME	Go to Sleep Time: _____	

BLOOD PRESSURE & WEIGHT

Time	SYS/DIA	Pulse

WEIGHT: _____

NOTES/SCHEDULE

7 am	
8 am	
9 am	
10 am	
11 am	
12 am	
1 pm	
2 pm	
3 pm	
4 pm	
5 pm	
6 pm	
7 pm	
8 pm	

EXERCISE & ACTIVITY LOG

	Time/Duration	Intensity/Calories

DATE: _____   SU | MO | TU | WE | TH | FR | SA   **Month/Week:** _____

FOOD, NUTRITION & MEDS

	Carbs	Sugar	Fiber	Protein	Fat	Calories
BREAKFAST Time: _____ Meds/Insulin: _____						
Breakfast Total						
SNACK 1 Time: _____ Meds/Insulin: _____						
Snack 1 Total						
LUNCH Time: _____ Meds/Insulin: _____						
Lunch Total						
SNACK 2 Time: _____ Meds/Insulin: _____						
Snack 2 Total						
DINNER Time: _____ Meds/Insulin: _____						
Dinner Total						
Total Nutrition for the Day						

Water Consumption ⬜ ⬜ ⬜ ⬜ ⬜ ⬜ ⬜ ⬜ ⬜ ⬜ _____

EXERCISE & ACTIVITY LOG

	Time/Duration	Intensity/Calories

BLOOD SUGAR LOG

	Blood Sugar Level	
	Before	**After**
WAKING UP Time: _____	Sleep Hrs: _____ Fast. Hrs: _____	
BREAKFAST		
SNACK 1		
LUNCH		
SNACK 2		
DINNER		
BEDTIME	Go to Sleep Time: _____	

BLOOD PRESSURE & WEIGHT

Time	SYS/DIA	Pulse
WEIGHT: _____		

NOTES/SCHEDULE

7 am	
8 am	
9 am	
10 am	
11 am	
12 am	
1 pm	
2 pm	
3 pm	
4 pm	
5 pm	
6 pm	
7 pm	
8 pm	

DATE: _____ SU | MO | TU | WE | TH | FR | SA   **Month/Week:** _____

FOOD, NUTRITION & MEDS

	Carbs	Sugar	Fiber	Protein	Fat	Calories
BREAKFAST Time: _____ Meds/Insulin: _____						
Breakfast Total						
SNACK 1 Time: _____ Meds/Insulin: _____						
Snack 1 Total						
LUNCH Time: _____ Meds/Insulin: _____						
Lunch Total						
SNACK 2 Time: _____ Meds/Insulin: _____						
Snack 2 Total						
DINNER Time: _____ Meds/Insulin: _____						
Dinner Total						
Total Nutrition for the Day						

Water Consumption ⬜⬜⬜⬜⬜⬜⬜⬜⬜⬜ _____

EXERCISE & ACTIVITY LOG

	Time/Duration	Intensity/Calories

BLOOD SUGAR LOG

	Blood Sugar Level	
	Before	**After**
WAKING UP Time: _____	Sleep Hrs: _____ Fast. Hrs: _____	
BREAKFAST		
SNACK 1		
LUNCH		
SNACK 2		
DINNER		
BEDTIME	Go to Sleep Time: _____	

BLOOD PRESSURE & WEIGHT

Time	SYS/DIA	Pulse

WEIGHT: _____

NOTES/SCHEDULE

7 am	
8 am	
9 am	
10 am	
11 am	
12 am	
1 pm	
2 pm	
3 pm	
4 pm	
5 pm	
6 pm	
7 pm	
8 pm	

DATE: _____ SU | MO | TU | WE | TH | FR | SA   **Month/Week:** _____

FOOD, NUTRITION & MEDS

	Carbs	Sugar	Fiber	Protein	Fat	Calories
BREAKFAST Time: _____ Meds/Insulin: _____						
Breakfast Total						
SNACK 1 Time: _____ Meds/Insulin: _____						
Snack 1 Total						
LUNCH Time: _____ Meds/Insulin: _____						
Lunch Total						
SNACK 2 Time: _____ Meds/Insulin: _____						
Snack 2 Total						
DINNER Time: _____ Meds/Insulin: _____						
Dinner Total						
Total Nutrition for the Day						

Water Consumption ⬜⬜⬜⬜⬜⬜⬜⬜⬜⬜ _____

BLOOD SUGAR LOG

	Blood Sugar Level	
	Before	**After**
WAKING UP Time: _____	Sleep Hrs: _____ Fast. Hrs: _____	
BREAKFAST		
SNACK 1		
LUNCH		
SNACK 2		
DINNER		
BEDTIME	Go to Sleep Time: _____	

BLOOD PRESSURE & WEIGHT

Time	SYS/DIA	Pulse
WEIGHT: _____		

NOTES/SCHEDULE

7 am	
8 am	
9 am	
10 am	
11 am	
12 am	
1 pm	
2 pm	
3 pm	
4 pm	
5 pm	
6 pm	
7 pm	
8 pm	

EXERCISE & ACTIVITY LOG

	Time/Duration	Intensity/Calories

DATE: _____ SU | MO | TU | WE | TH | FR | SA   **Month/Week:** _____

FOOD, NUTRITION & MEDS

	Carbs	Sugar	Fiber	Protein	Fat	Calories
BREAKFAST Time: _____ Meds/Insulin: _____						
Breakfast Total						
SNACK 1 Time: _____ Meds/Insulin: _____						
Snack 1 Total						
LUNCH Time: _____ Meds/Insulin: _____						
Lunch Total						
SNACK 2 Time: _____ Meds/Insulin: _____						
Snack 2 Total						
DINNER Time: _____ Meds/Insulin: _____						
Dinner Total						
Total Nutrition for the Day						

Water Consumption 🥛 🥛 🥛 🥛 🥛 🥛 🥛 🥛 🥛 🥛 _____

EXERCISE & ACTIVITY LOG

	Time/Duration	Intensity/Calories

BLOOD SUGAR LOG

	Blood Sugar Level	
	Before	**After**
WAKING UP Time: _____	Sleep Hrs: _____ Fast. Hrs: _____	
BREAKFAST		
SNACK 1		
LUNCH		
SNACK 2		
DINNER		
BEDTIME	Go to Sleep Time: _____	

BLOOD PRESSURE & WEIGHT

Time	SYS/DIA	Pulse
WEIGHT: _____		

NOTES/SCHEDULE

7 am	
8 am	
9 am	
10 am	
11 am	
12 am	
1 pm	
2 pm	
3 pm	
4 pm	
5 pm	
6 pm	
7 pm	
8 pm	

DATE: _____ SU | MO | TU | WE | TH | FR | SA   **Month/Week:** _____

FOOD, NUTRITION & MEDS

	Carbs	Sugar	Fiber	Protein	Fat	Calories
BREAKFAST Time: _____ Meds/Insulin: _____						
Breakfast Total						
SNACK 1 Time: _____ Meds/Insulin: _____						
Snack 1 Total						
LUNCH Time: _____ Meds/Insulin: _____						
Lunch Total						
SNACK 2 Time: _____ Meds/Insulin: _____						
Snack 2 Total						
DINNER Time: _____ Meds/Insulin: _____						
Dinner Total						
Total Nutrition for the Day						

Water Consumption ⎕ ⎕ ⎕ ⎕ ⎕ ⎕ ⎕ ⎕ ⎕ ⎕ _____

EXERCISE & ACTIVITY LOG

	Time/Duration	Intensity/Calories

BLOOD SUGAR LOG

	Blood Sugar Level	
	Before	**After**
WAKING UP Time: _____	Sleep Hrs: _____ Fast. Hrs: _____	
BREAKFAST		
SNACK 1		
LUNCH		
SNACK 2		
DINNER		
BEDTIME	Go to Sleep Time: _____	

BLOOD PRESSURE & WEIGHT

Time	SYS/DIA	Pulse

WEIGHT: _____

NOTES/SCHEDULE

7 am	
8 am	
9 am	
10 am	
11 am	
12 am	
1 pm	
2 pm	
3 pm	
4 pm	
5 pm	
6 pm	
7 pm	
8 pm	

DATE: _____ SU | MO | TU | WE | TH | FR | SA   **Month/Week:** _____

FOOD, NUTRITION & MEDS

	Carbs	Sugar	Fiber	Protein	Fat	Calories
BREAKFAST Time: _____ Meds/Insulin: _____						
Breakfast Total						
SNACK 1 Time: _____ Meds/Insulin: _____						
Snack 1 Total						
LUNCH Time: _____ Meds/Insulin: _____						
Lunch Total						
SNACK 2 Time: _____ Meds/Insulin: _____						
Snack 2 Total						
DINNER Time: _____ Meds/Insulin: _____						
Dinner Total						
Total Nutrition for the Day						

Water Consumption ▯ ▯ ▯ ▯ ▯ ▯ ▯ ▯ ▯ ▯ _____

BLOOD SUGAR LOG

	Blood Sugar Level	
	Before	**After**
WAKING UP Time: _____	Sleep Hrs: _____ Fast. Hrs: _____	
BREAKFAST		
SNACK 1		
LUNCH		
SNACK 2		
DINNER		
BEDTIME	Go to Sleep Time: _____	

BLOOD PRESSURE & WEIGHT

Time	SYS/DIA	Pulse
WEIGHT: _____		

NOTES/SCHEDULE

7 am	
8 am	
9 am	
10 am	
11 am	
12 am	
1 pm	
2 pm	
3 pm	
4 pm	
5 pm	
6 pm	
7 pm	
8 pm	

EXERCISE & ACTIVITY LOG

	Time/Duration	Intensity/Calories

DATE: _____   SU | MO | TU | WE | TH | FR | SA   **Month/Week:** _____

FOOD, NUTRITION & MEDS

	Carbs	Sugar	Fiber	Protein	Fat	Calories
BREAKFAST Time: _____ Meds/Insulin: _____						
Breakfast Total						
SNACK 1 Time: _____ Meds/Insulin: _____						
Snack 1 Total						
LUNCH Time: _____ Meds/Insulin: _____						
Lunch Total						
SNACK 2 Time: _____ Meds/Insulin: _____						
Snack 2 Total						
DINNER Time: _____ Meds/Insulin: _____						
Dinner Total						
Total Nutrition for the Day						

Water Consumption ⬜ ⬜ ⬜ ⬜ ⬜ ⬜ ⬜ ⬜ ⬜ _____

BLOOD SUGAR LOG

	Blood Sugar Level	
	Before	**After**
WAKING UP Time: _____	Sleep Hrs: _____ Fast. Hrs: _____	
BREAKFAST		
SNACK 1		
LUNCH		
SNACK 2		
DINNER		
BEDTIME	Go to Sleep Time: _____	

BLOOD PRESSURE & WEIGHT

Time	SYS/DIA	Pulse

WEIGHT: _____

NOTES/SCHEDULE

7 am	
8 am	
9 am	
10 am	
11 am	
12 am	
1 pm	
2 pm	
3 pm	
4 pm	
5 pm	
6 pm	
7 pm	
8 pm	

EXERCISE & ACTIVITY LOG

	Time/Duration	Intensity/Calories

DATE: _____   SU | MO | TU | WE | TH | FR | SA   **Month/Week:** _____

FOOD, NUTRITION & MEDS

	Carbs	Sugar	Fiber	Protein	Fat	Calories
BREAKFAST Time: _____ Meds/Insulin: _____						
Breakfast Total						
SNACK 1 Time: _____ Meds/Insulin: _____						
Snack 1 Total						
LUNCH Time: _____ Meds/Insulin: _____						
Lunch Total						
SNACK 2 Time: _____ Meds/Insulin: _____						
Snack 2 Total						
DINNER Time: _____ Meds/Insulin: _____						
Dinner Total						
Total Nutrition for the Day						

Water Consumption ⬛⬛⬛⬛⬛⬛⬛⬛⬛ _____

BLOOD SUGAR LOG

	Blood Sugar Level	
	Before	**After**
WAKING UP Time: _____	Sleep Hrs: _____ Fast. Hrs: _____	
BREAKFAST		
SNACK 1		
LUNCH		
SNACK 2		
DINNER		
BEDTIME	Go to Sleep Time: _____	

BLOOD PRESSURE & WEIGHT

Time	SYS/DIA	Pulse
WEIGHT: _____		

NOTES/SCHEDULE

7 am	
8 am	
9 am	
10 am	
11 am	
12 am	
1 pm	
2 pm	
3 pm	
4 pm	
5 pm	
6 pm	
7 pm	
8 pm	

EXERCISE & ACTIVITY LOG

	Time/Duration	Intensity/Calories

DATE: _____ SU | MO | TU | WE | TH | FR | SA   **Month/Week:** _____

FOOD, NUTRITION & MEDS

	Carbs	Sugar	Fiber	Protein	Fat	Calories
BREAKFAST Time: _____ Meds/Insulin: _____						
Breakfast Total						
SNACK 1 Time: _____ Meds/Insulin: _____						
Snack 1 Total						
LUNCH Time: _____ Meds/Insulin: _____						
Lunch Total						
SNACK 2 Time: _____ Meds/Insulin: _____						
Snack 2 Total						
DINNER Time: _____ Meds/Insulin: _____						
Dinner Total						
Total Nutrition for the Day						

Water Consumption ☐ ☐ ☐ ☐ ☐ ☐ ☐ ☐ ☐ ☐ _____

EXERCISE & ACTIVITY LOG

	Time/Duration	Intensity/Calories

BLOOD SUGAR LOG

	Blood Sugar Level	
	Before	**After**
WAKING UP Time: _____	Sleep Hrs: _____ Fast. Hrs: _____	
BREAKFAST		
SNACK 1		
LUNCH		
SNACK 2		
DINNER		
BEDTIME	Go to Sleep Time: _____	

BLOOD PRESSURE & WEIGHT

Time	SYS/DIA	Pulse

WEIGHT: _____

NOTES/SCHEDULE

7 am	
8 am	
9 am	
10 am	
11 am	
12 am	
1 pm	
2 pm	
3 pm	
4 pm	
5 pm	
6 pm	
7 pm	
8 pm	

DATE: _____   SU | MO | TU | WE | TH | FR | SA   **Month/Week:** _____

FOOD, NUTRITION & MEDS

	Carbs	Sugar	Fiber	Protein	Fat	Calories
BREAKFAST Time: _____ Meds/Insulin: _____						
Breakfast Total						
SNACK 1 Time: _____ Meds/Insulin: _____						
Snack 1 Total						
LUNCH Time: _____ Meds/Insulin: _____						
Lunch Total						
SNACK 2 Time: _____ Meds/Insulin: _____						
Snack 2 Total						
DINNER Time: _____ Meds/Insulin: _____						
Dinner Total						
Total Nutrition for the Day						

Water Consumption ⬜⬜⬜⬜⬜⬜⬜⬜⬜ _____

EXERCISE & ACTIVITY LOG

	Time/Duration	Intensity/Calories

BLOOD SUGAR LOG

	Blood Sugar Level	
	Before	**After**
WAKING UP Time: _____	Sleep Hrs: _____ Fast. Hrs: _____	
BREAKFAST		
SNACK 1		
LUNCH		
SNACK 2		
DINNER		
BEDTIME	Go to Sleep Time: _____	

BLOOD PRESSURE & WEIGHT

Time	SYS/DIA	Pulse

WEIGHT: _____

NOTES/SCHEDULE

7 am	
8 am	
9 am	
10 am	
11 am	
12 am	
1 pm	
2 pm	
3 pm	
4 pm	
5 pm	
6 pm	
7 pm	
8 pm	

DATE: _____   SU | MO | TU | WE | TH | FR | SA   **Month/Week:** _____

FOOD, NUTRITION & MEDS

	Carbs	Sugar	Fiber	Protein	Fat	Calories
BREAKFAST Time: _____ Meds/Insulin: _____						
Breakfast Total						
SNACK 1 Time: _____ Meds/Insulin: _____						
Snack 1 Total						
LUNCH Time: _____ Meds/Insulin: _____						
Lunch Total						
SNACK 2 Time: _____ Meds/Insulin: _____						
Snack 2 Total						
DINNER Time: _____ Meds/Insulin: _____						
Dinner Total						
Total Nutrition for the Day						

Water Consumption 🥛🥛🥛🥛🥛🥛🥛🥛🥛🥛 _____

EXERCISE & ACTIVITY LOG

	Time/Duration	Intensity/Calories

BLOOD SUGAR LOG

	Blood Sugar Level	
	Before	**After**
WAKING UP Time: _____	Sleep Hrs: _____ Fast. Hrs: _____	
BREAKFAST		
SNACK 1		
LUNCH		
SNACK 2		
DINNER		
BEDTIME	Go to Sleep Time: _____	

BLOOD PRESSURE & WEIGHT

Time	SYS/DIA	Pulse
WEIGHT: _____		

NOTES/SCHEDULE

7 am	
8 am	
9 am	
10 am	
11 am	
12 am	
1 pm	
2 pm	
3 pm	
4 pm	
5 pm	
6 pm	
7 pm	
8 pm	

DATE: _____   SU | MO | TU | WE | TH | FR | SA   **Month/Week:** _____

FOOD, NUTRITION & MEDS

	Carbs	Sugar	Fiber	Protein	Fat	Calories
BREAKFAST Time: _____ Meds/Insulin: _____						
Breakfast Total						
SNACK 1 Time: _____ Meds/Insulin: _____						
Snack 1 Total						
LUNCH Time: _____ Meds/Insulin: _____						
Lunch Total						
SNACK 2 Time: _____ Meds/Insulin: _____						
Snack 2 Total						
DINNER Time: _____ Meds/Insulin: _____						
Dinner Total						
Total Nutrition for the Day						

Water Consumption 🥛🥛🥛🥛🥛 🥛🥛🥛🥛🥛 _____

EXERCISE & ACTIVITY LOG

	Time/Duration	Intensity/Calories

BLOOD SUGAR LOG

	Blood Sugar Level	
	Before	**After**
WAKING UP Time: _____	Sleep Hrs: _____ Fast. Hrs: _____	
BREAKFAST		
SNACK 1		
LUNCH		
SNACK 2		
DINNER		
BEDTIME	Go to Sleep Time: _____	

BLOOD PRESSURE & WEIGHT

Time	SYS/DIA	Pulse

WEIGHT: _____

NOTES/SCHEDULE

7 am	
8 am	
9 am	
10 am	
11 am	
12 am	
1 pm	
2 pm	
3 pm	
4 pm	
5 pm	
6 pm	
7 pm	
8 pm	

DATE: _____   SU | MO | TU | WE | TH | FR | SA   **Month/Week:** _____

FOOD, NUTRITION & MEDS

		Carbs	Sugar	Fiber	Protein	Fat	Calories
BREAKFAST Time: _____ Meds/Insulin: _____							
	Breakfast Total						
SNACK 1 Time: _____ Meds/Insulin: _____							
	Snack 1 Total						
LUNCH Time: _____ Meds/Insulin: _____							
	Lunch Total						
SNACK 2 Time: _____ Meds/Insulin: _____							
	Snack 2 Total						
DINNER Time: _____ Meds/Insulin: _____							
	Dinner Total						
	Total Nutrition for the Day						

Water Consumption ⬜ ⬜ ⬜ ⬜ ⬜ ⬜ ⬜ ⬜ ⬜ ⬜   _____

BLOOD SUGAR LOG

	Blood Sugar Level	
	Before	**After**
WAKING UP Time: _____	Sleep Hrs: _____ Fast. Hrs: _____	
BREAKFAST		
SNACK 1		
LUNCH		
SNACK 2		
DINNER		
BEDTIME	Go to Sleep Time: _____	

BLOOD PRESSURE & WEIGHT

Time	SYS/DIA	Pulse
WEIGHT: _____		

NOTES/SCHEDULE

7 am	
8 am	
9 am	
10 am	
11 am	
12 am	
1 pm	
2 pm	
3 pm	
4 pm	
5 pm	
6 pm	
7 pm	
8 pm	

EXERCISE & ACTIVITY LOG

	Time/Duration	Intensity/Calories

DATE: _____ SU | MO | TU | WE | TH | FR | SA   **Month/Week:** _____

FOOD, NUTRITION & MEDS

	Carbs	Sugar	Fiber	Protein	Fat	Calories
BREAKFAST Time: _____ Meds/Insulin: _____						
Breakfast Total						
SNACK 1 Time: _____ Meds/Insulin: _____						
Snack 1 Total						
LUNCH Time: _____ Meds/Insulin: _____						
Lunch Total						
SNACK 2 Time: _____ Meds/Insulin: _____						
Snack 2 Total						
DINNER Time: _____ Meds/Insulin: _____						
Dinner Total						
Total Nutrition for the Day						

Water Consumption 🥤🥤🥤🥤🥤🥤🥤🥤🥤🥤 _____

EXERCISE & ACTIVITY LOG

	Time/Duration	Intensity/Calories

BLOOD SUGAR LOG

	Blood Sugar Level	
	Before	**After**
WAKING UP Time: _____	Sleep Hrs: _____ Fast. Hrs: _____	
BREAKFAST		
SNACK 1		
LUNCH		
SNACK 2		
DINNER		
BEDTIME	Go to Sleep Time: _____	

BLOOD PRESSURE & WEIGHT

Time	SYS/DIA	Pulse

WEIGHT: _____

NOTES/SCHEDULE

7 am	
8 am	
9 am	
10 am	
11 am	
12 am	
1 pm	
2 pm	
3 pm	
4 pm	
5 pm	
6 pm	
7 pm	
8 pm	

DATE: _____   SU | MO | TU | WE | TH | FR | SA   **Month/Week:** _____

FOOD, NUTRITION & MEDS

	Carbs	Sugar	Fiber	Protein	Fat	Calories
BREAKFAST Time: _____ Meds/Insulin: _____						
Breakfast Total						
SNACK 1 Time: _____ Meds/Insulin: _____						
Snack 1 Total						
LUNCH Time: _____ Meds/Insulin: _____						
Lunch Total						
SNACK 2 Time: _____ Meds/Insulin: _____						
Snack 2 Total						
DINNER Time: _____ Meds/Insulin: _____						
Dinner Total						
Total Nutrition for the Day						

Water Consumption ▢▢▢▢▢▢▢▢▢ _____

EXERCISE & ACTIVITY LOG

	Time/Duration	Intensity/Calories

BLOOD SUGAR LOG

	Blood Sugar Level	
	Before	**After**
WAKING UP Time: _____	Sleep Hrs: _____ Fast. Hrs: _____	
BREAKFAST		
SNACK 1		
LUNCH		
SNACK 2		
DINNER		
BEDTIME	Go to Sleep Time: _____	

BLOOD PRESSURE & WEIGHT

Time	SYS/DIA	Pulse

WEIGHT: _____

NOTES/SCHEDULE

7 am	
8 am	
9 am	
10 am	
11 am	
12 am	
1 pm	
2 pm	
3 pm	
4 pm	
5 pm	
6 pm	
7 pm	
8 pm	

DATE: _____ SU | MO | TU | WE | TH | FR | SA   **Month/Week:** _____

FOOD, NUTRITION & MEDS

	Carbs	Sugar	Fiber	Protein	Fat	Calories
BREAKFAST Time: _____ Meds/Insulin: _____						
Breakfast Total						
SNACK 1 Time: _____ Meds/Insulin: _____						
Snack 1 Total						
LUNCH Time: _____ Meds/Insulin: _____						
Lunch Total						
SNACK 2 Time: _____ Meds/Insulin: _____						
Snack 2 Total						
DINNER Time: _____ Meds/Insulin: _____						
Dinner Total						
Total Nutrition for the Day						

Water Consumption ☐ ☐ ☐ ☐ ☐ ☐ ☐ ☐ ☐ ☐ _____

EXERCISE & ACTIVITY LOG

	Time/Duration	Intensity/Calories

BLOOD SUGAR LOG

	Blood Sugar Level	
	Before	**After**
WAKING UP Time: _____	Sleep Hrs: _____ Fast. Hrs: _____	
BREAKFAST		
SNACK 1		
LUNCH		
SNACK 2		
DINNER		
BEDTIME	Go to Sleep Time: _____	

BLOOD PRESSURE & WEIGHT

Time	SYS/DIA	Pulse
WEIGHT: _____		

NOTES/SCHEDULE

7 am	
8 am	
9 am	
10 am	
11 am	
12 am	
1 pm	
2 pm	
3 pm	
4 pm	
5 pm	
6 pm	
7 pm	
8 pm	

DATE: _____ SU | MO | TU | WE | TH | FR | SA   **Month/Week:** _____

FOOD, NUTRITION & MEDS

	Carbs	Sugar	Fiber	Protein	Fat	Calories
BREAKFAST Time: _____ Meds/Insulin: _____						
Breakfast Total						
SNACK 1 Time: _____ Meds/Insulin: _____						
Snack 1 Total						
LUNCH Time: _____ Meds/Insulin: _____						
Lunch Total						
SNACK 2 Time: _____ Meds/Insulin: _____						
Snack 2 Total						
DINNER Time: _____ Meds/Insulin: _____						
Dinner Total						
Total Nutrition for the Day						

Water Consumption ⬜⬜⬜⬜⬜⬜⬜⬜⬜⬜ _____

EXERCISE & ACTIVITY LOG

	Time/Duration	Intensity/Calories

BLOOD SUGAR LOG

	Blood Sugar Level	
	Before	**After**
WAKING UP Time: _____	Sleep Hrs: _____ Fast. Hrs: _____	
BREAKFAST		
SNACK 1		
LUNCH		
SNACK 2		
DINNER		
BEDTIME	Go to Sleep Time: _____	

BLOOD PRESSURE & WEIGHT

Time	SYS/DIA	Pulse
WEIGHT: _____		

NOTES/SCHEDULE

7 am	
8 am	
9 am	
10 am	
11 am	
12 am	
1 pm	
2 pm	
3 pm	
4 pm	
5 pm	
6 pm	
7 pm	
8 pm	

DATE: _____   SU | MO | TU | WE | TH | FR | SA   **Month/Week:** _____

FOOD, NUTRITION & MEDS

	Carbs	Sugar	Fiber	Protein	Fat	Calories
BREAKFAST Time: _____ Meds/Insulin: _____						
Breakfast Total						
SNACK 1 Time: _____ Meds/Insulin: _____						
Snack 1 Total						
LUNCH Time: _____ Meds/Insulin: _____						
Lunch Total						
SNACK 2 Time: _____ Meds/Insulin: _____						
Snack 2 Total						
DINNER Time: _____ Meds/Insulin: _____						
Dinner Total						
Total Nutrition for the Day						

Water Consumption ▯ ▯ ▯ ▯ ▯ ▯ ▯ ▯ ▯ ▯   _____

EXERCISE & ACTIVITY LOG

	Time/Duration	Intensity/Calories

BLOOD SUGAR LOG

	Blood Sugar Level	
	Before	After
WAKING UP Time: _____	Sleep Hrs: _____ Fast. Hrs: _____	
BREAKFAST		
SNACK 1		
LUNCH		
SNACK 2		
DINNER		
BEDTIME	Go to Sleep Time: _____	

BLOOD PRESSURE & WEIGHT

Time	SYS/DIA	Pulse
WEIGHT: _____		

NOTES/SCHEDULE

7 am	
8 am	
9 am	
10 am	
11 am	
12 am	
1 pm	
2 pm	
3 pm	
4 pm	
5 pm	
6 pm	
7 pm	
8 pm	

DATE: _____ SU | MO | TU | WE | TH | FR | SA   **Month/Week:** _____

FOOD, NUTRITION & MEDS

	Carbs	Sugar	Fiber	Protein	Fat	Calories
BREAKFAST Time: _____ Meds/Insulin: _____						
Breakfast Total						
SNACK 1 Time: _____ Meds/Insulin: _____						
Snack 1 Total						
LUNCH Time: _____ Meds/Insulin: _____						
Lunch Total						
SNACK 2 Time: _____ Meds/Insulin: _____						
Snack 2 Total						
DINNER Time: _____ Meds/Insulin: _____						
Dinner Total						
Total Nutrition for the Day						

Water Consumption ☐ ☐ ☐ ☐ ☐ ☐ ☐ ☐ ☐ ☐ _____

EXERCISE & ACTIVITY LOG

	Time/Duration	Intensity/Calories

BLOOD SUGAR LOG

	Blood Sugar Level	
	Before	**After**
WAKING UP Time: _____	Sleep Hrs: _____ Fast. Hrs: _____	
BREAKFAST		
SNACK 1		
LUNCH		
SNACK 2		
DINNER		
BEDTIME	Go to Sleep Time: _____	

BLOOD PRESSURE & WEIGHT

Time	SYS/DIA	Pulse
WEIGHT: _____		

NOTES/SCHEDULE

7 am	
8 am	
9 am	
10 am	
11 am	
12 am	
1 pm	
2 pm	
3 pm	
4 pm	
5 pm	
6 pm	
7 pm	
8 pm	

DATE: _____ SU | MO | TU | WE | TH | FR | SA **Month/Week:** _____

FOOD, NUTRITION & MEDS

	Carbs	Sugar	Fiber	Protein	Fat	Calories
BREAKFAST Time: _____ Meds/Insulin: _____						
Breakfast Total						
SNACK 1 Time: _____ Meds/Insulin: _____						
Snack 1 Total						
LUNCH Time: _____ Meds/Insulin: _____						
Lunch Total						
SNACK 2 Time: _____ Meds/Insulin: _____						
Snack 2 Total						
DINNER Time: _____ Meds/Insulin: _____						
Dinner Total						
Total Nutrition for the Day						

Water Consumption ⬚⬚⬚⬚⬚⬚⬚⬚⬚⬚ _____

EXERCISE & ACTIVITY LOG

	Time/Duration	Intensity/Calories

BLOOD SUGAR LOG

	Blood Sugar Level	
	Before	**After**
WAKING UP Time: _____	Sleep Hrs: _____ Fast. Hrs: _____	
BREAKFAST		
SNACK 1		
LUNCH		
SNACK 2		
DINNER		
BEDTIME	Go to Sleep Time: _____	

BLOOD PRESSURE & WEIGHT

Time	SYS/DIA	Pulse
WEIGHT: _____		

NOTES/SCHEDULE

7 am	
8 am	
9 am	
10 am	
11 am	
12 am	
1 pm	
2 pm	
3 pm	
4 pm	
5 pm	
6 pm	
7 pm	
8 pm	

DATE: _____   SU | MO | TU | WE | TH | FR | SA   **Month/Week:** _____

FOOD, NUTRITION & MEDS

		Carbs	Sugar	Fiber	Protein	Fat	Calories
BREAKFAST Time: _____ Meds/Insulin: _____							
Breakfast Total							
SNACK 1 Time: _____ Meds/Insulin: _____							
Snack 1 Total							
LUNCH Time: _____ Meds/Insulin: _____							
Lunch Total							
SNACK 2 Time: _____ Meds/Insulin: _____							
Snack 2 Total							
DINNER Time: _____ Meds/Insulin: _____							
Dinner Total							
Total Nutrition for the Day							

Water Consumption ⬜⬜⬜⬜⬜⬜⬜⬜⬜⬜ _____

BLOOD SUGAR LOG

	Blood Sugar Level	
	Before	**After**
WAKING UP Time: _____	Sleep Hrs: _____ Fast. Hrs: _____	
BREAKFAST		
SNACK 1		
LUNCH		
SNACK 2		
DINNER		
BEDTIME	Go to Sleep Time: _____	

BLOOD PRESSURE & WEIGHT

Time	SYS/DIA	Pulse

WEIGHT: _____

NOTES/SCHEDULE

7 am	
8 am	
9 am	
10 am	
11 am	
12 am	
1 pm	
2 pm	
3 pm	
4 pm	
5 pm	
6 pm	
7 pm	
8 pm	

EXERCISE & ACTIVITY LOG

	Time/Duration	Intensity/Calories

DATE: _____ SU | MO | TU | WE | TH | FR | SA **Month/Week:** _____

FOOD, NUTRITION & MEDS

	Carbs	Sugar	Fiber	Protein	Fat	Calories
BREAKFAST Time: _____ Meds/Insulin: _____						
Breakfast Total						
SNACK 1 Time: _____ Meds/Insulin: _____						
Snack 1 Total						
LUNCH Time: _____ Meds/Insulin: _____						
Lunch Total						
SNACK 2 Time: _____ Meds/Insulin: _____						
Snack 2 Total						
DINNER Time: _____ Meds/Insulin: _____						
Dinner Total						
Total Nutrition for the Day						

Water Consumption 🥛🥛🥛🥛🥛🥛🥛🥛🥛🥛 _____

EXERCISE & ACTIVITY LOG

	Time/Duration	Intensity/Calories

BLOOD SUGAR LOG

	Blood Sugar Level	
	Before	**After**
WAKING UP Time: _____	Sleep Hrs: _____ Fast. Hrs: _____	
BREAKFAST		
SNACK 1		
LUNCH		
SNACK 2		
DINNER		
BEDTIME	Go to Sleep Time: _____	

BLOOD PRESSURE & WEIGHT

Time	SYS/DIA	Pulse

WEIGHT: _____

NOTES/SCHEDULE

7 am	
8 am	
9 am	
10 am	
11 am	
12 am	
1 pm	
2 pm	
3 pm	
4 pm	
5 pm	
6 pm	
7 pm	
8 pm	

DATE: _____ SU | MO | TU | WE | TH | FR | SA   **Month/Week:** _____

FOOD, NUTRITION & MEDS

	Carbs	Sugar	Fiber	Protein	Fat	Calories
BREAKFAST Time: _____ Meds/Insulin: _____						
Breakfast Total						
SNACK 1 Time: _____ Meds/Insulin: _____						
Snack 1 Total						
LUNCH Time: _____ Meds/Insulin: _____						
Lunch Total						
SNACK 2 Time: _____ Meds/Insulin: _____						
Snack 2 Total						
DINNER Time: _____ Meds/Insulin: _____						
Dinner Total						
Total Nutrition for the Day						

Water Consumption ☐ ☐ ☐ ☐ ☐ ☐ ☐ ☐ ☐ ☐ _____

EXERCISE & ACTIVITY LOG

	Time/Duration	Intensity/Calories

BLOOD SUGAR LOG

	Blood Sugar Level	
	Before	**After**
WAKING UP Time: _____	Sleep Hrs: _____ Fast. Hrs: _____	
BREAKFAST		
SNACK 1		
LUNCH		
SNACK 2		
DINNER		
BEDTIME	Go to Sleep Time: _____	

BLOOD PRESSURE & WEIGHT

Time	SYS/DIA	Pulse
WEIGHT: _____		

NOTES/SCHEDULE

7 am	
8 am	
9 am	
10 am	
11 am	
12 am	
1 pm	
2 pm	
3 pm	
4 pm	
5 pm	
6 pm	
7 pm	
8 pm	

Month/Week: _____

FOOD, NUTRITION & MEDS

	Carbs	Sugar	Fiber	Protein	Fat	Calories
BREAKFAST Time: _____ Meds/Insulin: _____						
Breakfast Total						
SNACK 1 Time: _____ Meds/Insulin: _____						
Snack 1 Total						
LUNCH Time: _____ Meds/Insulin: _____						
Lunch Total						
SNACK 2 Time: _____ Meds/Insulin: _____						
Snack 2 Total						
DINNER Time: _____ Meds/Insulin: _____						
Dinner Total						
Total Nutrition for the Day						

Water Consumption ▯ ▯ ▯ ▯ ▯ ▯ ▯ ▯ ▯ ▯ _____

EXERCISE & ACTIVITY LOG

	Time/Duration	Intensity/Calories

BLOOD SUGAR LOG

	Blood Sugar Level	
	Before	**After**
WAKING UP Time: _____	Sleep Hrs: _____ Fast. Hrs: _____	
BREAKFAST		
SNACK 1		
LUNCH		
SNACK 2		
DINNER		
BEDTIME	Go to Sleep Time: _____	

BLOOD PRESSURE & WEIGHT

Time	SYS/DIA	Pulse

WEIGHT: _____

NOTES/SCHEDULE

7 am	
8 am	
9 am	
10 am	
11 am	
12 am	
1 pm	
2 pm	
3 pm	
4 pm	
5 pm	
6 pm	
7 pm	
8 pm	

DATE: _____ SU | MO | TU | WE | TH | FR | SA   **Month/Week:** _____

FOOD, NUTRITION & MEDS

	Carbs	Sugar	Fiber	Protein	Fat	Calories
BREAKFAST Time: _____ Meds/Insulin: _____						
Breakfast Total						
SNACK 1 Time: _____ Meds/Insulin: _____						
Snack 1 Total						
LUNCH Time: _____ Meds/Insulin: _____						
Lunch Total						
SNACK 2 Time: _____ Meds/Insulin: _____						
Snack 2 Total						
DINNER Time: _____ Meds/Insulin: _____						
Dinner Total						
Total Nutrition for the Day						

Water Consumption ☐ ☐ ☐ ☐ ☐ ☐ ☐ ☐ ☐ ☐ _____

EXERCISE & ACTIVITY LOG

	Time/Duration	Intensity/Calories

BLOOD SUGAR LOG

	Blood Sugar Level	
	Before	**After**
WAKING UP Time: _____	Sleep Hrs: _____ Fast. Hrs: _____	
BREAKFAST		
SNACK 1		
LUNCH		
SNACK 2		
DINNER		
BEDTIME	Go to Sleep Time: _____	

BLOOD PRESSURE & WEIGHT

Time	SYS/DIA	Pulse

WEIGHT: _____

NOTES/SCHEDULE

7 am	
8 am	
9 am	
10 am	
11 am	
12 am	
1 pm	
2 pm	
3 pm	
4 pm	
5 pm	
6 pm	
7 pm	
8 pm	

FOOD, NUTRITION & MEDS

		Carbs	Sugar	Fiber	Protein	Fat	Calories
BREAKFAST Time: _____ Meds/Insulin: _____							
	Breakfast Total						
SNACK 1 Time: _____ Meds/Insulin: _____							
	Snack 1 Total						
LUNCH Time: _____ Meds/Insulin: _____							
	Lunch Total						
SNACK 2 Time: _____ Meds/Insulin: _____							
	Snack 2 Total						
DINNER Time: _____ Meds/Insulin: _____							
	Dinner Total						
	Total Nutrition for the Day						

Water Consumption ⬜ ⬜ ⬜ ⬜ ⬜ ⬜ ⬜ ⬜ ⬜ ⬜ _____

EXERCISE & ACTIVITY LOG

	Time/Duration	Intensity/Calories

BLOOD SUGAR LOG

		Blood Sugar Level	
		Before	**After**
WAKING UP Time: _____	Sleep Hrs: _____ Fast. Hrs: _____		
BREAKFAST			
SNACK 1			
LUNCH			
SNACK 2			
DINNER			
BEDTIME	Go to Sleep Time: _____		

BLOOD PRESSURE & WEIGHT

Time	SYS/DIA	Pulse

WEIGHT: _____

NOTES/SCHEDULE

7 am	
8 am	
9 am	
10 am	
11 am	
12 am	
1 pm	
2 pm	
3 pm	
4 pm	
5 pm	
6 pm	
7 pm	
8 pm	

DATE: _____   SU | MO | TU | WE | TH | FR | SA   **Month/Week:** _____

FOOD, NUTRITION & MEDS

	Carbs	Sugar	Fiber	Protein	Fat	Calories
BREAKFAST Time: _____ Meds/Insulin: _____						
Breakfast Total						
SNACK 1 Time: _____ Meds/Insulin: _____						
Snack 1 Total						
LUNCH Time: _____ Meds/Insulin: _____						
Lunch Total						
SNACK 2 Time: _____ Meds/Insulin: _____						
Snack 2 Total						
DINNER Time: _____ Meds/Insulin: _____						
Dinner Total						
Total Nutrition for the Day						

Water Consumption   ⬜⬜⬜⬜⬜⬜⬜⬜⬜   _____

BLOOD SUGAR LOG

	Blood Sugar Level	
	Before	**After**
WAKING UP Time: _____	Sleep Hrs: _____ Fast. Hrs: _____	
BREAKFAST		
SNACK 1		
LUNCH		
SNACK 2		
DINNER		
BEDTIME	Go to Sleep Time: _____	

BLOOD PRESSURE & WEIGHT

Time	SYS/DIA	Pulse

WEIGHT: _____

NOTES/SCHEDULE

7 am	
8 am	
9 am	
10 am	
11 am	
12 am	
1 pm	
2 pm	
3 pm	
4 pm	
5 pm	
6 pm	
7 pm	
8 pm	

EXERCISE & ACTIVITY LOG

	Time/Duration	Intensity/Calories

DATE: _____   SU | MO | TU | WE | TH | FR | SA   **Month/Week:** _____

FOOD, NUTRITION & MEDS

	Carbs	Sugar	Fiber	Protein	Fat	Calories
BREAKFAST Time: _____ Meds/Insulin: _____						
Breakfast Total						
SNACK 1 Time: _____ Meds/Insulin: _____						
Snack 1 Total						
LUNCH Time: _____ Meds/Insulin: _____						
Lunch Total						
SNACK 2 Time: _____ Meds/Insulin: _____						
Snack 2 Total						
DINNER Time: _____ Meds/Insulin: _____						
Dinner Total						
Total Nutrition for the Day						

Water Consumption   ▯ ▯ ▯ ▯ ▯ ▯ ▯ ▯ ▯   _____

EXERCISE & ACTIVITY LOG

	Time/Duration	Intensity/Calories

BLOOD SUGAR LOG

	Blood Sugar Level	
	Before	**After**
WAKING UP Time: _____	Sleep Hrs: _____ Fast. Hrs: _____	
BREAKFAST		
SNACK 1		
LUNCH		
SNACK 2		
DINNER		
BEDTIME	Go to Sleep Time: _____	

BLOOD PRESSURE & WEIGHT

Time	SYS/DIA	Pulse

WEIGHT: _____

NOTES/SCHEDULE

7 am	
8 am	
9 am	
10 am	
11 am	
12 am	
1 pm	
2 pm	
3 pm	
4 pm	
5 pm	
6 pm	
7 pm	
8 pm	

DATE: _____ SU | MO | TU | WE | TH | FR | SA   **Month/Week:** _____

FOOD, NUTRITION & MEDS

	Carbs	Sugar	Fiber	Protein	Fat	Calories
BREAKFAST Time: _____ Meds/Insulin: _____						
Breakfast Total						
SNACK 1 Time: _____ Meds/Insulin: _____						
Snack 1 Total						
LUNCH Time: _____ Meds/Insulin: _____						
Lunch Total						
SNACK 2 Time: _____ Meds/Insulin: _____						
Snack 2 Total						
DINNER Time: _____ Meds/Insulin: _____						
Dinner Total						
Total Nutrition for the Day						

Water Consumption ⬜⬜⬜⬜⬜⬜⬜⬜⬜⬜ _____

EXERCISE & ACTIVITY LOG

	Time/Duration	Intensity/Calories

BLOOD SUGAR LOG

	Blood Sugar Level	
	Before	**After**
WAKING UP Time: _____	Sleep Hrs: _____ Fast. Hrs: _____	
BREAKFAST		
SNACK 1		
LUNCH		
SNACK 2		
DINNER		
BEDTIME	Go to Sleep Time: _____	

BLOOD PRESSURE & WEIGHT

Time	SYS/DIA	Pulse

WEIGHT: _____

NOTES/SCHEDULE

7 am	
8 am	
9 am	
10 am	
11 am	
12 am	
1 pm	
2 pm	
3 pm	
4 pm	
5 pm	
6 pm	
7 pm	
8 pm	

DATE: _____ SU | MO | TU | WE | TH | FR | SA   **Month/Week:** _____

FOOD, NUTRITION & MEDS

	Carbs	Sugar	Fiber	Protein	Fat	Calories
BREAKFAST Time: _____ Meds/Insulin: _____						
Breakfast Total						
SNACK 1 Time: _____ Meds/Insulin: _____						
Snack 1 Total						
LUNCH Time: _____ Meds/Insulin: _____						
Lunch Total						
SNACK 2 Time: _____ Meds/Insulin: _____						
Snack 2 Total						
DINNER Time: _____ Meds/Insulin: _____						
Dinner Total						
Total Nutrition for the Day						

Water Consumption ⬜ ⬜ ⬜ ⬜ ⬜ ⬜ ⬜ ⬜ ⬜ ⬜ _____

EXERCISE & ACTIVITY LOG

	Time/Duration	Intensity/Calories

BLOOD SUGAR LOG

	Blood Sugar Level	
	Before	**After**
WAKING UP Time: _____	Sleep Hrs: _____ Fast. Hrs: _____	
BREAKFAST		
SNACK 1		
LUNCH		
SNACK 2		
DINNER		
BEDTIME	Go to Sleep Time: _____	

BLOOD PRESSURE & WEIGHT

Time	SYS/DIA	Pulse
WEIGHT: _____		

NOTES/SCHEDULE

7 am	
8 am	
9 am	
10 am	
11 am	
12 am	
1 pm	
2 pm	
3 pm	
4 pm	
5 pm	
6 pm	
7 pm	
8 pm	

DATE: _____ SU | MO | TU | WE | TH | FR | SA   **Month/Week:** _____

FOOD, NUTRITION & MEDS

	Carbs	Sugar	Fiber	Protein	Fat	Calories
BREAKFAST Time: _____ Meds/Insulin: _____						
Breakfast Total						
SNACK 1 Time: _____ Meds/Insulin: _____						
Snack 1 Total						
LUNCH Time: _____ Meds/Insulin: _____						
Lunch Total						
SNACK 2 Time: _____ Meds/Insulin: _____						
Snack 2 Total						
DINNER Time: _____ Meds/Insulin: _____						
Dinner Total						
Total Nutrition for the Day						

Water Consumption ⬚ ⬚ ⬚ ⬚ ⬚ ⬚ ⬚ ⬚ ⬚ ⬚ _____

BLOOD SUGAR LOG

	Blood Sugar Level	
	Before	**After**
WAKING UP Time: _____	Sleep Hrs: _____ Fast. Hrs: _____	
BREAKFAST		
SNACK 1		
LUNCH		
SNACK 2		
DINNER		
BEDTIME	Go to Sleep Time: _____	

BLOOD PRESSURE & WEIGHT

Time	SYS/DIA	Pulse
WEIGHT: _____		

NOTES/SCHEDULE

7 am	
8 am	
9 am	
10 am	
11 am	
12 am	
1 pm	
2 pm	
3 pm	
4 pm	
5 pm	
6 pm	
7 pm	
8 pm	

EXERCISE & ACTIVITY LOG

	Time/Duration	Intensity/Calories

DATE: _____ SU | MO | TU | WE | TH | FR | SA   **Month/Week:** _____

FOOD, NUTRITION & MEDS

	Carbs	Sugar	Fiber	Protein	Fat	Calories
BREAKFAST Time: _____ Meds/Insulin: _____						
Breakfast Total						
SNACK 1 Time: _____ Meds/Insulin: _____						
Snack 1 Total						
LUNCH Time: _____ Meds/Insulin: _____						
Lunch Total						
SNACK 2 Time: _____ Meds/Insulin: _____						
Snack 2 Total						
DINNER Time: _____ Meds/Insulin: _____						
Dinner Total						
Total Nutrition for the Day						

Water Consumption 🥤🥤🥤🥤🥤🥤🥤🥤🥤🥤 _____

EXERCISE & ACTIVITY LOG

	Time/Duration	Intensity/Calories

BLOOD SUGAR LOG

	Blood Sugar Level	
	Before	**After**
WAKING UP Time: _____	Sleep Hrs: _____ Fast. Hrs: _____	
BREAKFAST		
SNACK 1		
LUNCH		
SNACK 2		
DINNER		
BEDTIME	Go to Sleep Time: _____	

BLOOD PRESSURE & WEIGHT

Time	SYS/DIA	Pulse

WEIGHT: _____

NOTES/SCHEDULE

7 am	
8 am	
9 am	
10 am	
11 am	
12 am	
1 pm	
2 pm	
3 pm	
4 pm	
5 pm	
6 pm	
7 pm	
8 pm	

DATE: _____   SU | MO | TU | WE | TH | FR | SA   **Month/Week:** _____

FOOD, NUTRITION & MEDS

	Carbs	Sugar	Fiber	Protein	Fat	Calories
BREAKFAST Time: _____ Meds/Insulin: _____						
Breakfast Total						
SNACK 1 Time: _____ Meds/Insulin: _____						
Snack 1 Total						
LUNCH Time: _____ Meds/Insulin: _____						
Lunch Total						
SNACK 2 Time: _____ Meds/Insulin: _____						
Snack 2 Total						
DINNER Time: _____ Meds/Insulin: _____						
Dinner Total						
Total Nutrition for the Day						

Water Consumption ▢ ▢ ▢ ▢ ▢ ▢ ▢ ▢ ▢ ▢   _____

EXERCISE & ACTIVITY LOG

	Time/Duration	Intensity/Calories

BLOOD SUGAR LOG

	Blood Sugar Level	
	Before	**After**
WAKING UP Time: _____	Sleep Hrs: _____ Fast. Hrs: _____	
BREAKFAST		
SNACK 1		
LUNCH		
SNACK 2		
DINNER		
BEDTIME	Go to Sleep Time: _____	

BLOOD PRESSURE & WEIGHT

Time	SYS/DIA	Pulse
WEIGHT: _____		

NOTES/SCHEDULE

7 am	
8 am	
9 am	
10 am	
11 am	
12 am	
1 pm	
2 pm	
3 pm	
4 pm	
5 pm	
6 pm	
7 pm	
8 pm	

DATE: _____ SU | MO | TU | WE | TH | FR | SA   **Month/Week:** _____

FOOD, NUTRITION & MEDS

	Carbs	Sugar	Fiber	Protein	Fat	Calories
BREAKFAST Time: _____ Meds/Insulin: _____						
Breakfast Total						
SNACK 1 Time: _____ Meds/Insulin: _____						
Snack 1 Total						
LUNCH Time: _____ Meds/Insulin: _____						
Lunch Total						
SNACK 2 Time: _____ Meds/Insulin: _____						
Snack 2 Total						
DINNER Time: _____ Meds/Insulin: _____						
Dinner Total						
Total Nutrition for the Day						

Water Consumption ⬜ ⬜ ⬜ ⬜ ⬜ ⬜ ⬜ ⬜ ⬜ ⬜ _____

EXERCISE & ACTIVITY LOG

	Time/Duration	Intensity/Calories

BLOOD SUGAR LOG

	Blood Sugar Level	
	Before	After
WAKING UP Time: _____	Sleep Hrs: _____ Fast. Hrs: _____	
BREAKFAST		
SNACK 1		
LUNCH		
SNACK 2		
DINNER		
BEDTIME	Go to Sleep Time: _____	

BLOOD PRESSURE & WEIGHT

Time	SYS/DIA	Pulse

WEIGHT: _____

NOTES/SCHEDULE

7 am	
8 am	
9 am	
10 am	
11 am	
12 am	
1 pm	
2 pm	
3 pm	
4 pm	
5 pm	
6 pm	
7 pm	
8 pm	

DATE: _____   SU | MO | TU | WE | TH | FR | SA   **Month/Week:** _____

FOOD, NUTRITION & MEDS

	Carbs	Sugar	Fiber	Protein	Fat	Calories
BREAKFAST Time: _____ Meds/Insulin: _____						
Breakfast Total						
SNACK 1 Time: _____ Meds/Insulin: _____						
Snack 1 Total						
LUNCH Time: _____ Meds/Insulin: _____						
Lunch Total						
SNACK 2 Time: _____ Meds/Insulin: _____						
Snack 2 Total						
DINNER Time: _____ Meds/Insulin: _____						
Dinner Total						
Total Nutrition for the Day						

Water Consumption ☐ ☐ ☐ ☐ ☐ ☐ ☐ ☐ ☐ ☐ _____

EXERCISE & ACTIVITY LOG

	Time/Duration	Intensity/Calories

BLOOD SUGAR LOG

	Blood Sugar Level	
	Before	**After**
WAKING UP Time: _____ Sleep Hrs: _____ Fast. Hrs: _____		
BREAKFAST		
SNACK 1		
LUNCH		
SNACK 2		
DINNER		
BEDTIME Go to Sleep Time: _____		

BLOOD PRESSURE & WEIGHT

Time	SYS/DIA	Pulse
WEIGHT: _____		

NOTES/SCHEDULE

7 am	
8 am	
9 am	
10 am	
11 am	
12 am	
1 pm	
2 pm	
3 pm	
4 pm	
5 pm	
6 pm	
7 pm	
8 pm	

DATE: _____ SU | MO | TU | WE | TH | FR | SA   **Month/Week:** _____

FOOD, NUTRITION & MEDS

	Carbs	Sugar	Fiber	Protein	Fat	Calories
BREAKFAST Time: _____ Meds/Insulin: _____						
Breakfast Total						
SNACK 1 Time: _____ Meds/Insulin: _____						
Snack 1 Total						
LUNCH Time: _____ Meds/Insulin: _____						
Lunch Total						
SNACK 2 Time: _____ Meds/Insulin: _____						
Snack 2 Total						
DINNER Time: _____ Meds/Insulin: _____						
Dinner Total						
Total Nutrition for the Day						

Water Consumption ⎕ ⎕ ⎕ ⎕ ⎕ ⎕ ⎕ ⎕ ⎕ ⎕ _____

EXERCISE & ACTIVITY LOG

	Time/Duration	Intensity/Calories

BLOOD SUGAR LOG

	Blood Sugar Level	
	Before	**After**
WAKING UP Time: _____	Sleep Hrs: _____ Fast. Hrs: _____	
BREAKFAST		
SNACK 1		
LUNCH		
SNACK 2		
DINNER		
BEDTIME	Go to Sleep Time: _____	

BLOOD PRESSURE & WEIGHT

Time	SYS/DIA	Pulse
WEIGHT: _____		

NOTES/SCHEDULE

7 am	
8 am	
9 am	
10 am	
11 am	
12 am	
1 pm	
2 pm	
3 pm	
4 pm	
5 pm	
6 pm	
7 pm	
8 pm	

DATE: _____   SU | MO | TU | WE | TH | FR | SA   **Month/Week:** _____

FOOD, NUTRITION & MEDS

	Carbs	Sugar	Fiber	Protein	Fat	Calories
BREAKFAST Time: _____ Meds/Insulin: _____						
Breakfast Total						
SNACK 1 Time: _____ Meds/Insulin: _____						
Snack 1 Total						
LUNCH Time: _____ Meds/Insulin: _____						
Lunch Total						
SNACK 2 Time: _____ Meds/Insulin: _____						
Snack 2 Total						
DINNER Time: _____ Meds/Insulin: _____						
Dinner Total						
Total Nutrition for the Day						

Water Consumption ⬛⬛⬛⬛⬛⬛⬛⬛⬛⬛ _____

BLOOD SUGAR LOG

	Blood Sugar Level	
	Before	**After**
WAKING UP Time: _____ Sleep Hrs: _____ Fast. Hrs: _____		
BREAKFAST		
SNACK 1		
LUNCH		
SNACK 2		
DINNER		
BEDTIME Go to Sleep Time: _____		

BLOOD PRESSURE & WEIGHT

Time	SYS/DIA	Pulse
WEIGHT: _____		

NOTES/SCHEDULE

7 am	
8 am	
9 am	
10 am	
11 am	
12 am	
1 pm	
2 pm	
3 pm	
4 pm	
5 pm	
6 pm	
7 pm	
8 pm	

EXERCISE & ACTIVITY LOG

	Time/Duration	Intensity/Calories

DATE: _____ SU | MO | TU | WE | TH | FR | SA   **Month/Week:** _____

FOOD, NUTRITION & MEDS

	Carbs	Sugar	Fiber	Protein	Fat	Calories
BREAKFAST Time: _____ Meds/Insulin: _____						
Breakfast Total						
SNACK 1 Time: _____ Meds/Insulin: _____						
Snack 1 Total						
LUNCH Time: _____ Meds/Insulin: _____						
Lunch Total						
SNACK 2 Time: _____ Meds/Insulin: _____						
Snack 2 Total						
DINNER Time: _____ Meds/Insulin: _____						
Dinner Total						
Total Nutrition for the Day						

Water Consumption ⬜ ⬜ ⬜ ⬜ ⬜ ⬜ ⬜ ⬜ ⬜ ⬜ _____

EXERCISE & ACTIVITY LOG

	Time/Duration	Intensity/Calories

BLOOD SUGAR LOG

	Blood Sugar Level	
	Before	**After**
WAKING UP Time: _____	Sleep Hrs: _____ Fast. Hrs: _____	
BREAKFAST		
SNACK 1		
LUNCH		
SNACK 2		
DINNER		
BEDTIME	Go to Sleep Time: _____	

BLOOD PRESSURE & WEIGHT

Time	SYS/DIA	Pulse

WEIGHT: _____

NOTES/SCHEDULE

7 am	
8 am	
9 am	
10 am	
11 am	
12 am	
1 pm	
2 pm	
3 pm	
4 pm	
5 pm	
6 pm	
7 pm	
8 pm	

DATE: _____ SU | MO | TU | WE | TH | FR | SA   **Month/Week:** _____

FOOD, NUTRITION & MEDS

	Carbs	Sugar	Fiber	Protein	Fat	Calories
BREAKFAST Time: _____ Meds/Insulin: _____						
Breakfast Total						
SNACK 1 Time: _____ Meds/Insulin: _____						
Snack 1 Total						
LUNCH Time: _____ Meds/Insulin: _____						
Lunch Total						
SNACK 2 Time: _____ Meds/Insulin: _____						
Snack 2 Total						
DINNER Time: _____ Meds/Insulin: _____						
Dinner Total						
Total Nutrition for the Day						

Water Consumption ⬜ ⬜ ⬜ ⬜ ⬜ ⬜ ⬜ ⬜ ⬜ ⬜   _____

EXERCISE & ACTIVITY LOG

	Time/Duration	Intensity/Calories

BLOOD SUGAR LOG

	Blood Sugar Level	
	Before	**After**
WAKING UP Time: _____	Sleep Hrs: _____ Fast. Hrs: _____	
BREAKFAST		
SNACK 1		
LUNCH		
SNACK 2		
DINNER		
BEDTIME	Go to Sleep Time: _____	

BLOOD PRESSURE & WEIGHT

Time	SYS/DIA	Pulse
WEIGHT: _____		

NOTES/SCHEDULE

7 am	
8 am	
9 am	
10 am	
11 am	
12 am	
1 pm	
2 pm	
3 pm	
4 pm	
5 pm	
6 pm	
7 pm	
8 pm	

DATE: _____ SU | MO | TU | WE | TH | FR | SA   **Month/Week:** _____

FOOD, NUTRITION & MEDS

	Carbs	Sugar	Fiber	Protein	Fat	Calories
BREAKFAST Time: _____ Meds/Insulin: _____						
Breakfast Total						
SNACK 1 Time: _____ Meds/Insulin: _____						
Snack 1 Total						
LUNCH Time: _____ Meds/Insulin: _____						
Lunch Total						
SNACK 2 Time: _____ Meds/Insulin: _____						
Snack 2 Total						
DINNER Time: _____ Meds/Insulin: _____						
Dinner Total						
Total Nutrition for the Day						

Water Consumption ⬜⬜⬜⬜⬜⬜⬜⬜⬜⬜ _____

BLOOD SUGAR LOG

	Blood Sugar Level	
	Before	**After**
WAKING UP Time: _____	Sleep Hrs: _____ Fast. Hrs: _____	
BREAKFAST		
SNACK 1		
LUNCH		
SNACK 2		
DINNER		
BEDTIME	Go to Sleep Time: _____	

BLOOD PRESSURE & WEIGHT

Time	SYS/DIA	Pulse
WEIGHT: _____		

NOTES/SCHEDULE

7 am	
8 am	
9 am	
10 am	
11 am	
12 am	
1 pm	
2 pm	
3 pm	
4 pm	
5 pm	
6 pm	
7 pm	
8 pm	

EXERCISE & ACTIVITY LOG

	Time/Duration	Intensity/Calories

DATE: _____ SU | MO | TU | WE | TH | FR | SA   **Month/Week:** _____

FOOD, NUTRITION & MEDS

	Carbs	Sugar	Fiber	Protein	Fat	Calories
BREAKFAST Time: _____ Meds/Insulin: _____						
Breakfast Total						
SNACK 1 Time: _____ Meds/Insulin: _____						
Snack 1 Total						
LUNCH Time: _____ Meds/Insulin: _____						
Lunch Total						
SNACK 2 Time: _____ Meds/Insulin: _____						
Snack 2 Total						
DINNER Time: _____ Meds/Insulin: _____						
Dinner Total						
Total Nutrition for the Day						

Water Consumption 🥛🥛🥛🥛🥛🥛🥛🥛🥛🥛 _____

EXERCISE & ACTIVITY LOG

	Time/Duration	Intensity/Calories

BLOOD SUGAR LOG

	Blood Sugar Level	
	Before	**After**
WAKING UP Time: _____	Sleep Hrs: _____ Fast. Hrs: _____	
BREAKFAST		
SNACK 1		
LUNCH		
SNACK 2		
DINNER		
BEDTIME	Go to Sleep Time: _____	

BLOOD PRESSURE & WEIGHT

Time	SYS/DIA	Pulse
WEIGHT: _____		

NOTES/SCHEDULE

7 am	
8 am	
9 am	
10 am	
11 am	
12 am	
1 pm	
2 pm	
3 pm	
4 pm	
5 pm	
6 pm	
7 pm	
8 pm	

DATE: _____ SU | MO | TU | WE | TH | FR | SA   **Month/Week:** _____

FOOD, NUTRITION & MEDS

	Carbs	Sugar	Fiber	Protein	Fat	Calories
BREAKFAST Time: _____ Meds/Insulin: _____						
Breakfast Total						
SNACK 1 Time: _____ Meds/Insulin: _____						
Snack 1 Total						
LUNCH Time: _____ Meds/Insulin: _____						
Lunch Total						
SNACK 2 Time: _____ Meds/Insulin: _____						
Snack 2 Total						
DINNER Time: _____ Meds/Insulin: _____						
Dinner Total						
Total Nutrition for the Day						

Water Consumption 🥛🥛🥛🥛🥛🥛🥛🥛🥛🥛 _____

EXERCISE & ACTIVITY LOG

	Time/Duration	Intensity/Calories

BLOOD SUGAR LOG

	Blood Sugar Level	
	Before	**After**
WAKING UP Time: _____	Sleep Hrs: _____ Fast. Hrs: _____	
BREAKFAST		
SNACK 1		
LUNCH		
SNACK 2		
DINNER		
BEDTIME	Go to Sleep Time: _____	

BLOOD PRESSURE & WEIGHT

Time	SYS/DIA	Pulse
WEIGHT: _____		

NOTES/SCHEDULE

7 am	
8 am	
9 am	
10 am	
11 am	
12 am	
1 pm	
2 pm	
3 pm	
4 pm	
5 pm	
6 pm	
7 pm	
8 pm	

DATE: _____ SU | MO | TU | WE | TH | FR | SA   **Month/Week:** _____

FOOD, NUTRITION & MEDS

	Carbs	Sugar	Fiber	Protein	Fat	Calories
BREAKFAST Time: _____ Meds/Insulin: _____						
Breakfast Total						
SNACK 1 Time: _____ Meds/Insulin: _____						
Snack 1 Total						
LUNCH Time: _____ Meds/Insulin: _____						
Lunch Total						
SNACK 2 Time: _____ Meds/Insulin: _____						
Snack 2 Total						
DINNER Time: _____ Meds/Insulin: _____						
Dinner Total						
Total Nutrition for the Day						

Water Consumption ▯ ▯ ▯ ▯ ▯ ▯ ▯ ▯ ▯ ▯   _____

BLOOD SUGAR LOG

	Blood Sugar Level	
	Before	**After**
WAKING UP Time: _____	Sleep Hrs: _____ Fast. Hrs: _____	
BREAKFAST		
SNACK 1		
LUNCH		
SNACK 2		
DINNER		
BEDTIME	Go to Sleep Time: _____	

BLOOD PRESSURE & WEIGHT

Time	SYS/DIA	Pulse

WEIGHT: _____

NOTES/SCHEDULE

7 am	
8 am	
9 am	
10 am	
11 am	
12 am	
1 pm	
2 pm	
3 pm	
4 pm	
5 pm	
6 pm	
7 pm	
8 pm	

EXERCISE & ACTIVITY LOG

	Time/Duration	Intensity/Calories

DATE: _____ SU | MO | TU | WE | TH | FR | SA

Month/Week: _____

FOOD, NUTRITION & MEDS

	Carbs	Sugar	Fiber	Protein	Fat	Calories
BREAKFAST Time: _____ Meds/Insulin: _____						
Breakfast Total						
SNACK 1 Time: _____ Meds/Insulin: _____						
Snack 1 Total						
LUNCH Time: _____ Meds/Insulin: _____						
Lunch Total						
SNACK 2 Time: _____ Meds/Insulin: _____						
Snack 2 Total						
DINNER Time: _____ Meds/Insulin: _____						
Dinner Total						
Total Nutrition for the Day						

Water Consumption ⬜ ⬜ ⬜ ⬜ ⬜ ⬜ ⬜ ⬜ ⬜ _____

EXERCISE & ACTIVITY LOG

	Time/Duration	Intensity/Calories

BLOOD SUGAR LOG

	Blood Sugar Level	
	Before	**After**
WAKING UP Time: _____	Sleep Hrs: _____ Fast. Hrs: _____	
BREAKFAST		
SNACK 1		
LUNCH		
SNACK 2		
DINNER		
BEDTIME	Go to Sleep Time: _____	

BLOOD PRESSURE & WEIGHT

Time	SYS/DIA	Pulse

WEIGHT: _____

NOTES/SCHEDULE

7 am	
8 am	
9 am	
10 am	
11 am	
12 am	
1 pm	
2 pm	
3 pm	
4 pm	
5 pm	
6 pm	
7 pm	
8 pm	

DATE: _____ SU | MO | TU | WE | TH | FR | SA   **Month/Week:** _____

FOOD, NUTRITION & MEDS

	Carbs	Sugar	Fiber	Protein	Fat	Calories
BREAKFAST Time: _____ Meds/Insulin: _____						
Breakfast Total						
SNACK 1 Time: _____ Meds/Insulin: _____						
Snack 1 Total						
LUNCH Time: _____ Meds/Insulin: _____						
Lunch Total						
SNACK 2 Time: _____ Meds/Insulin: _____						
Snack 2 Total						
DINNER Time: _____ Meds/Insulin: _____						
Dinner Total						
Total Nutrition for the Day						

Water Consumption ⬜⬜⬜⬜⬜⬜⬜⬜⬜⬜ _____

BLOOD SUGAR LOG

	Blood Sugar Level	
	Before	**After**
WAKING UP Time: _____ Sleep Hrs: _____ Fast. Hrs: _____		
BREAKFAST		
SNACK 1		
LUNCH		
SNACK 2		
DINNER		
BEDTIME Go to Sleep Time: _____		

BLOOD PRESSURE & WEIGHT

Time	SYS/DIA	Pulse

WEIGHT: _____

NOTES/SCHEDULE

7 am	
8 am	
9 am	
10 am	
11 am	
12 am	
1 pm	
2 pm	
3 pm	
4 pm	
5 pm	
6 pm	
7 pm	
8 pm	

EXERCISE & ACTIVITY LOG

	Time/Duration	Intensity/Calories

DATE: _____ SU | MO | TU | WE | TH | FR | SA   **Month/Week:** _____

FOOD, NUTRITION & MEDS

	Carbs	Sugar	Fiber	Protein	Fat	Calories
BREAKFAST Time: _____ Meds/Insulin: _____						
Breakfast Total						
SNACK 1 Time: _____ Meds/Insulin: _____						
Snack 1 Total						
LUNCH Time: _____ Meds/Insulin: _____						
Lunch Total						
SNACK 2 Time: _____ Meds/Insulin: _____						
Snack 2 Total						
DINNER Time: _____ Meds/Insulin: _____						
Dinner Total						
Total Nutrition for the Day						

Water Consumption 🥛🥛🥛🥛🥛🥛🥛🥛🥛🥛 _____

BLOOD SUGAR LOG

	Blood Sugar Level	
	Before	**After**
WAKING UP Time: _____	Sleep Hrs: _____ Fast. Hrs: _____	
BREAKFAST		
SNACK 1		
LUNCH		
SNACK 2		
DINNER		
BEDTIME	Go to Sleep Time: _____	

BLOOD PRESSURE & WEIGHT

Time	SYS/DIA	Pulse

WEIGHT: _____

NOTES/SCHEDULE

7 am	
8 am	
9 am	
10 am	
11 am	
12 am	
1 pm	
2 pm	
3 pm	
4 pm	
5 pm	
6 pm	
7 pm	
8 pm	

EXERCISE & ACTIVITY LOG

	Time/Duration	Intensity/Calories

DATE: _____   SU | MO | TU | WE | TH | FR | SA   **Month/Week:** _____

FOOD, NUTRITION & MEDS

	Carbs	Sugar	Fiber	Protein	Fat	Calories
BREAKFAST Time: _____ Meds/Insulin: _____						
Breakfast Total						
SNACK 1 Time: _____ Meds/Insulin: _____						
Snack 1 Total						
LUNCH Time: _____ Meds/Insulin: _____						
Lunch Total						
SNACK 2 Time: _____ Meds/Insulin: _____						
Snack 2 Total						
DINNER Time: _____ Meds/Insulin: _____						
Dinner Total						
Total Nutrition for the Day						

Water Consumption ⬜⬜⬜⬜⬜⬜⬜⬜⬜⬜ _____

BLOOD SUGAR LOG

	Blood Sugar Level	
	Before	**After**
WAKING UP Time: _____	Sleep Hrs: _____ Fast. Hrs: _____	
BREAKFAST		
SNACK 1		
LUNCH		
SNACK 2		
DINNER		
BEDTIME	Go to Sleep Time: _____	

BLOOD PRESSURE & WEIGHT

Time	SYS/DIA	Pulse
WEIGHT: _____		

NOTES/SCHEDULE

7 am	
8 am	
9 am	
10 am	
11 am	
12 am	
1 pm	
2 pm	
3 pm	
4 pm	
5 pm	
6 pm	
7 pm	
8 pm	

EXERCISE & ACTIVITY LOG

	Time/Duration	Intensity/Calories

DATE: _____   SU | MO | TU | WE | TH | FR | SA   **Month/Week:** _____

FOOD, NUTRITION & MEDS

BREAKFAST Time: _____ Meds/Insulin: _____	Carbs	Sugar	Fiber	Protein	Fat	Calories
Breakfast Total						

SNACK 1 Time: _____ Meds/Insulin: _____						
Snack 1 Total						

LUNCH Time: _____ Meds/Insulin: _____						
Lunch Total						

SNACK 2 Time: _____ Meds/Insulin: _____						
Snack 2 Total						

DINNER Time: _____ Meds/Insulin: _____						
Dinner Total						
Total Nutrition for the Day						

Water Consumption ▢ ▢ ▢ ▢ ▢ ▢ ▢ ▢ ▢ ▢ _____

EXERCISE & ACTIVITY LOG

	Time/Duration	Intensity/Calories

BLOOD SUGAR LOG

	Blood Sugar Level	
	Before	**After**
WAKING UP Time: _____	Sleep Hrs: _____ Fast. Hrs: _____	
BREAKFAST		
SNACK 1		
LUNCH		
SNACK 2		
DINNER		
BEDTIME	Go to Sleep Time: _____	

BLOOD PRESSURE & WEIGHT

Time	SYS/DIA	Pulse
WEIGHT: _____		

NOTES/SCHEDULE

7 am	
8 am	
9 am	
10 am	
11 am	
12 am	
1 pm	
2 pm	
3 pm	
4 pm	
5 pm	
6 pm	
7 pm	
8 pm	

DATE: _____ SU | MO | TU | WE | TH | FR | SA   Month/Week: _____

FOOD, NUTRITION & MEDS

	Carbs	Sugar	Fiber	Protein	Fat	Calories
BREAKFAST Time: _____ Meds/Insulin: _____						
Breakfast Total						
SNACK 1 Time: _____ Meds/Insulin: _____						
Snack 1 Total						
LUNCH Time: _____ Meds/Insulin: _____						
Lunch Total						
SNACK 2 Time: _____ Meds/Insulin: _____						
Snack 2 Total						
DINNER Time: _____ Meds/Insulin: _____						
Dinner Total						
Total Nutrition for the Day						

Water Consumption ⬜ ⬜ ⬜ ⬜ ⬜ ⬜ ⬜ ⬜ ⬜ ⬜ _____

EXERCISE & ACTIVITY LOG

	Time/Duration	Intensity/Calories

BLOOD SUGAR LOG

	Blood Sugar Level	
	Before	**After**
WAKING UP Time: _____	Sleep Hrs: _____ Fast. Hrs: _____	
BREAKFAST		
SNACK 1		
LUNCH		
SNACK 2		
DINNER		
BEDTIME	Go to Sleep Time: _____	

BLOOD PRESSURE & WEIGHT

Time	SYS/DIA	Pulse
WEIGHT: _____		

NOTES/SCHEDULE

7 am	
8 am	
9 am	
10 am	
11 am	
12 am	
1 pm	
2 pm	
3 pm	
4 pm	
5 pm	
6 pm	
7 pm	
8 pm	

DATE: _____   SU | MO | TU | WE | TH | FR | SA   **Month/Week:** _____

FOOD, NUTRITION & MEDS

	Carbs	Sugar	Fiber	Protein	Fat	Calories
BREAKFAST Time: _____ Meds/Insulin: _____						
Breakfast Total						
SNACK 1 Time: _____ Meds/Insulin: _____						
Snack 1 Total						
LUNCH Time: _____ Meds/Insulin: _____						
Lunch Total						
SNACK 2 Time: _____ Meds/Insulin: _____						
Snack 2 Total						
DINNER Time: _____ Meds/Insulin: _____						
Dinner Total						
Total Nutrition for the Day						

Water Consumption ⬜⬜⬜⬜⬜⬜⬜⬜⬜ _____

EXERCISE & ACTIVITY LOG

	Time/Duration	Intensity/Calories

BLOOD SUGAR LOG

	Blood Sugar Level	
	Before	**After**
WAKING UP Time: _____	Sleep Hrs: _____ Fast. Hrs: _____	
BREAKFAST		
SNACK 1		
LUNCH		
SNACK 2		
DINNER		
BEDTIME	Go to Sleep Time: _____	

BLOOD PRESSURE & WEIGHT

Time	SYS/DIA	Pulse

WEIGHT: _____

NOTES/SCHEDULE

7 am	
8 am	
9 am	
10 am	
11 am	
12 am	
1 pm	
2 pm	
3 pm	
4 pm	
5 pm	
6 pm	
7 pm	
8 pm	

DATE: _____   SU | MO | TU | WE | TH | FR | SA   **Month/Week:** _____

FOOD, NUTRITION & MEDS

	Carbs	Sugar	Fiber	Protein	Fat	Calories
BREAKFAST Time: _____ Meds/Insulin: _____						
Breakfast Total						
SNACK 1 Time: _____ Meds/Insulin: _____						
Snack 1 Total						
LUNCH Time: _____ Meds/Insulin: _____						
Lunch Total						
SNACK 2 Time: _____ Meds/Insulin: _____						
Snack 2 Total						
DINNER Time: _____ Meds/Insulin: _____						
Dinner Total						
Total Nutrition for the Day						

Water Consumption 🥛🥛🥛🥛🥛🥛🥛🥛🥛🥛 _____

EXERCISE & ACTIVITY LOG

	Time/Duration	Intensity/Calories

BLOOD SUGAR LOG

	Blood Sugar Level	
	Before	**After**
WAKING UP Time: _____	Sleep Hrs: _____ Fast. Hrs: _____	
BREAKFAST		
SNACK 1		
LUNCH		
SNACK 2		
DINNER		
BEDTIME	Go to Sleep Time: _____	

BLOOD PRESSURE & WEIGHT

Time	SYS/DIA	Pulse

WEIGHT: _____

NOTES/SCHEDULE

7 am	
8 am	
9 am	
10 am	
11 am	
12 am	
1 pm	
2 pm	
3 pm	
4 pm	
5 pm	
6 pm	
7 pm	
8 pm	

DATE: _____   SU | MO | TU | WE | TH | FR | SA

Month/Week: _____

FOOD, NUTRITION & MEDS

	Carbs	Sugar	Fiber	Protein	Fat	Calories
BREAKFAST Time: _____ Meds/Insulin: _____						
Breakfast Total						
SNACK 1 Time: _____ Meds/Insulin: _____						
Snack 1 Total						
LUNCH Time: _____ Meds/Insulin: _____						
Lunch Total						
SNACK 2 Time: _____ Meds/Insulin: _____						
Snack 2 Total						
DINNER Time: _____ Meds/Insulin: _____						
Dinner Total						
Total Nutrition for the Day						

Water Consumption ☐ ☐ ☐ ☐ ☐ ☐ ☐ ☐ ☐ _____

EXERCISE & ACTIVITY LOG

	Time/Duration	Intensity/Calories

BLOOD SUGAR LOG

	Blood Sugar Level	
	Before	**After**
WAKING UP Time: _____	Sleep Hrs: _____ Fast. Hrs: _____	
BREAKFAST		
SNACK 1		
LUNCH		
SNACK 2		
DINNER		
BEDTIME	Go to Sleep Time: _____	

BLOOD PRESSURE & WEIGHT

Time	SYS/DIA	Pulse

WEIGHT: _____

NOTES/SCHEDULE

7 am	
8 am	
9 am	
10 am	
11 am	
12 am	
1 pm	
2 pm	
3 pm	
4 pm	
5 pm	
6 pm	
7 pm	
8 pm	

DATE: _____ SU | MO | TU | WE | TH | FR | SA   **Month/Week:** _____

FOOD, NUTRITION & MEDS

	Carbs	Sugar	Fiber	Protein	Fat	Calories
BREAKFAST Time: _____ Meds/Insulin: _____						
Breakfast Total						
SNACK 1 Time: _____ Meds/Insulin: _____						
Snack 1 Total						
LUNCH Time: _____ Meds/Insulin: _____						
Lunch Total						
SNACK 2 Time: _____ Meds/Insulin: _____						
Snack 2 Total						
DINNER Time: _____ Meds/Insulin: _____						
Dinner Total						
Total Nutrition for the Day						

Water Consumption ⬚ ⬚ ⬚ ⬚ ⬚ ⬚ ⬚ ⬚ ⬚ ⬚ _____

EXERCISE & ACTIVITY LOG

	Time/Duration	Intensity/Calories

BLOOD SUGAR LOG

	Blood Sugar Level	
	Before	**After**
WAKING UP Time: _____	Sleep Hrs: _____ Fast. Hrs: _____	
BREAKFAST		
SNACK 1		
LUNCH		
SNACK 2		
DINNER		
BEDTIME	Go to Sleep Time: _____	

BLOOD PRESSURE & WEIGHT

Time	SYS/DIA	Pulse
WEIGHT: _____		

NOTES/SCHEDULE

7 am	
8 am	
9 am	
10 am	
11 am	
12 am	
1 pm	
2 pm	
3 pm	
4 pm	
5 pm	
6 pm	
7 pm	
8 pm	

DATE: _____ SU | MO | TU | WE | TH | FR | SA **Month/Week:** _____

FOOD, NUTRITION & MEDS

	Carbs	Sugar	Fiber	Protein	Fat	Calories

BREAKFAST Time: _____ Meds/Insulin: _____

Breakfast Total						

SNACK 1 Time: _____ Meds/Insulin: _____

Snack 1 Total						

LUNCH Time: _____ Meds/Insulin: _____

Lunch Total						

SNACK 2 Time: _____ Meds/Insulin: _____

Snack 2 Total						

DINNER Time: _____ Meds/Insulin: _____

Dinner Total						
Total Nutrition for the Day						

Water Consumption ☐ ☐ ☐ ☐ ☐ ☐ ☐ ☐ ☐ ☐ _____

EXERCISE & ACTIVITY LOG

	Time/Duration	Intensity/Calories

BLOOD SUGAR LOG

	Blood Sugar Level	
	Before	**After**
WAKING UP Time: _____	Sleep Hrs: _____ Fast. Hrs: _____	
BREAKFAST		
SNACK 1		
LUNCH		
SNACK 2		
DINNER		
BEDTIME	Go to Sleep Time: _____	

BLOOD PRESSURE & WEIGHT

Time	SYS/DIA	Pulse

WEIGHT: _____

NOTES/SCHEDULE

7 am	
8 am	
9 am	
10 am	
11 am	
12 am	
1 pm	
2 pm	
3 pm	
4 pm	
5 pm	
6 pm	
7 pm	
8 pm	

DATE: _____   SU | MO | TU | WE | TH | FR | SA   **Month/Week:** _____

FOOD, NUTRITION & MEDS

	Carbs	Sugar	Fiber	Protein	Fat	Calories
BREAKFAST Time: _____ Meds/Insulin: _____						
Breakfast Total						
SNACK 1 Time: _____ Meds/Insulin: _____						
Snack 1 Total						
LUNCH Time: _____ Meds/Insulin: _____						
Lunch Total						
SNACK 2 Time: _____ Meds/Insulin: _____						
Snack 2 Total						
DINNER Time: _____ Meds/Insulin: _____						
Dinner Total						
Total Nutrition for the Day						

Water Consumption   ▯ ▯ ▯ ▯ ▯ ▯ ▯ ▯ ▯ ▯   _____

BLOOD SUGAR LOG

	Blood Sugar Level	
	Before	**After**
WAKING UP Time: _____	Sleep Hrs: _____ Fast. Hrs: _____	
BREAKFAST		
SNACK 1		
LUNCH		
SNACK 2		
DINNER		
BEDTIME	Go to Sleep Time: _____	

BLOOD PRESSURE & WEIGHT

Time	SYS/DIA	Pulse

WEIGHT: _____

NOTES/SCHEDULE

7 am	
8 am	
9 am	
10 am	
11 am	
12 am	
1 pm	
2 pm	
3 pm	
4 pm	
5 pm	
6 pm	
7 pm	
8 pm	

EXERCISE & ACTIVITY LOG

	Time/Duration	Intensity/Calories

DATE: _____   SU | MO | TU | WE | TH | FR | SA   **Month/Week:** _____

FOOD, NUTRITION & MEDS

	Carbs	Sugar	Fiber	Protein	Fat	Calories
BREAKFAST Time: _____ Meds/Insulin: _____						
Breakfast Total						
SNACK 1 Time: _____ Meds/Insulin: _____						
Snack 1 Total						
LUNCH Time: _____ Meds/Insulin: _____						
Lunch Total						
SNACK 2 Time: _____ Meds/Insulin: _____						
Snack 2 Total						
DINNER Time: _____ Meds/Insulin: _____						
Dinner Total						
Total Nutrition for the Day						

Water Consumption ☐ ☐ ☐ ☐ ☐ ☐ ☐ ☐ ☐ ☐   _____

BLOOD SUGAR LOG

	Blood Sugar Level	
	Before	**After**
WAKING UP Time: _____	Sleep Hrs: _____ Fast. Hrs: _____	
BREAKFAST		
SNACK 1		
LUNCH		
SNACK 2		
DINNER		
BEDTIME	Go to Sleep Time: _____	

BLOOD PRESSURE & WEIGHT

Time	SYS/DIA	Pulse
WEIGHT: _____		

NOTES/SCHEDULE

7 am	
8 am	
9 am	
10 am	
11 am	
12 am	
1 pm	
2 pm	
3 pm	
4 pm	
5 pm	
6 pm	
7 pm	
8 pm	

EXERCISE & ACTIVITY LOG

	Time/Duration	Intensity/Calories

DATE: _____ SU | MO | TU | WE | TH | FR | SA   **Month/Week:** _____

FOOD, NUTRITION & MEDS

	Carbs	Sugar	Fiber	Protein	Fat	Calories
BREAKFAST Time: _____ Meds/Insulin: _____						
Breakfast Total						
SNACK 1 Time: _____ Meds/Insulin: _____						
Snack 1 Total						
LUNCH Time: _____ Meds/Insulin: _____						
Lunch Total						
SNACK 2 Time: _____ Meds/Insulin: _____						
Snack 2 Total						
DINNER Time: _____ Meds/Insulin: _____						
Dinner Total						
Total Nutrition for the Day						

Water Consumption ▢ ▢ ▢ ▢ ▢ ▢ ▢ ▢ ▢ ▢ _____

EXERCISE & ACTIVITY LOG

	Time/Duration	Intensity/Calories

BLOOD SUGAR LOG

	Blood Sugar Level	
	Before	**After**
WAKING UP Time: _____	Sleep Hrs: _____ Fast. Hrs: _____	
BREAKFAST		
SNACK 1		
LUNCH		
SNACK 2		
DINNER		
BEDTIME	Go to Sleep Time: _____	

BLOOD PRESSURE & WEIGHT

Time	SYS/DIA	Pulse
WEIGHT: _____		

NOTES/SCHEDULE

7 am	
8 am	
9 am	
10 am	
11 am	
12 am	
1 pm	
2 pm	
3 pm	
4 pm	
5 pm	
6 pm	
7 pm	
8 pm	

DATE: _____ SU | MO | TU | WE | TH | FR | SA

Month/Week: _____

FOOD, NUTRITION & MEDS

	Carbs	Sugar	Fiber	Protein	Fat	Calories
BREAKFAST Time: _____ Meds/Insulin: _____						
Breakfast Total						
SNACK 1 Time: _____ Meds/Insulin: _____						
Snack 1 Total						
LUNCH Time: _____ Meds/Insulin: _____						
Lunch Total						
SNACK 2 Time: _____ Meds/Insulin: _____						
Snack 2 Total						
DINNER Time: _____ Meds/Insulin: _____						
Dinner Total						
Total Nutrition for the Day						

Water Consumption ▢ ▢ ▢ ▢ ▢ ▢ ▢ ▢ ▢ _____

BLOOD SUGAR LOG

	Blood Sugar Level	
	Before	**After**
WAKING UP Time: _____	Sleep Hrs: _____ Fast. Hrs: _____	
BREAKFAST		
SNACK 1		
LUNCH		
SNACK 2		
DINNER		
BEDTIME	Go to Sleep Time: _____	

BLOOD PRESSURE & WEIGHT

Time	SYS/DIA	Pulse
WEIGHT: _____		

NOTES/SCHEDULE

7 am	
8 am	
9 am	
10 am	
11 am	
12 am	
1 pm	
2 pm	
3 pm	
4 pm	
5 pm	
6 pm	
7 pm	
8 pm	

EXERCISE & ACTIVITY LOG

	Time/Duration	Intensity/Calories

DATE: _____   SU | MO | TU | WE | TH | FR | SA   **Month/Week:** _____

FOOD, NUTRITION & MEDS

	Carbs	Sugar	Fiber	Protein	Fat	Calories
BREAKFAST Time: _____ Meds/Insulin: _____						
Breakfast Total						
SNACK 1 Time: _____ Meds/Insulin: _____						
Snack 1 Total						
LUNCH Time: _____ Meds/Insulin: _____						
Lunch Total						
SNACK 2 Time: _____ Meds/Insulin: _____						
Snack 2 Total						
DINNER Time: _____ Meds/Insulin: _____						
Dinner Total						
Total Nutrition for the Day						

Water Consumption 🥛🥛🥛🥛🥛🥛🥛🥛🥛🥛 _____

BLOOD SUGAR LOG

	Blood Sugar Level	
	Before	**After**
WAKING UP Time: _____	Sleep Hrs: _____ Fast. Hrs: _____	
BREAKFAST		
SNACK 1		
LUNCH		
SNACK 2		
DINNER		
BEDTIME	Go to Sleep Time: _____	

BLOOD PRESSURE & WEIGHT

Time	SYS/DIA	Pulse
WEIGHT: _____		

NOTES/SCHEDULE

7 am	
8 am	
9 am	
10 am	
11 am	
12 am	
1 pm	
2 pm	
3 pm	
4 pm	
5 pm	
6 pm	
7 pm	
8 pm	

EXERCISE & ACTIVITY LOG

	Time/Duration	Intensity/Calories

DATE: _____ SU | MO | TU | WE | TH | FR | SA   **Month/Week:** _____

FOOD, NUTRITION & MEDS

BREAKFAST Time: _____ Meds/Insulin: _____	Carbs	Sugar	Fiber	Protein	Fat	Calories
Breakfast Total						

SNACK 1 Time: _____ Meds/Insulin: _____						
Snack 1 Total						

LUNCH Time: _____ Meds/Insulin: _____						
Lunch Total						

SNACK 2 Time: _____ Meds/Insulin: _____						
Snack 2 Total						

DINNER Time: _____ Meds/Insulin: _____						
Dinner Total						
Total Nutrition for the Day						

Water Consumption ▯▯▯▯▯ ▯▯▯▯▯ _____

EXERCISE & ACTIVITY LOG

	Time/Duration	Intensity/Calories

BLOOD SUGAR LOG

	Blood Sugar Level	
	Before	**After**
WAKING UP Time: _____	Sleep Hrs: _____ Fast. Hrs: _____	
BREAKFAST		
SNACK 1		
LUNCH		
SNACK 2		
DINNER		
BEDTIME	Go to Sleep Time: _____	

BLOOD PRESSURE & WEIGHT

Time	SYS/DIA	Pulse
WEIGHT: _____		

NOTES/SCHEDULE

7 am	
8 am	
9 am	
10 am	
11 am	
12 am	
1 pm	
2 pm	
3 pm	
4 pm	
5 pm	
6 pm	
7 pm	
8 pm	

DATE: _____ SU | MO | TU | WE | TH | FR | SA   **Month/Week:** _____

FOOD, NUTRITION & MEDS

	Carbs	Sugar	Fiber	Protein	Fat	Calories
BREAKFAST Time: _____ Meds/Insulin: _____						
Breakfast Total						
SNACK 1 Time: _____ Meds/Insulin: _____						
Snack 1 Total						
LUNCH Time: _____ Meds/Insulin: _____						
Lunch Total						
SNACK 2 Time: _____ Meds/Insulin: _____						
Snack 2 Total						
DINNER Time: _____ Meds/Insulin: _____						
Dinner Total						
Total Nutrition for the Day						

Water Consumption ☐ ☐ ☐ ☐ ☐ ☐ ☐ ☐ ☐ ☐ _____

BLOOD SUGAR LOG

	Blood Sugar Level	
	Before	**After**
WAKING UP Time: _____	Sleep Hrs: _____ Fast. Hrs: _____	
BREAKFAST		
SNACK 1		
LUNCH		
SNACK 2		
DINNER		
BEDTIME	Go to Sleep Time: _____	

BLOOD PRESSURE & WEIGHT

Time	SYS/DIA	Pulse
WEIGHT: _____		

NOTES/SCHEDULE

7 am	
8 am	
9 am	
10 am	
11 am	
12 am	
1 pm	
2 pm	
3 pm	
4 pm	
5 pm	
6 pm	
7 pm	
8 pm	

EXERCISE & ACTIVITY LOG

	Time/Duration	Intensity/Calories

DATE: _____ SU | MO | TU | WE | TH | FR | SA

Month/Week: _____

FOOD, NUTRITION & MEDS

	Carbs	Sugar	Fiber	Protein	Fat	Calories
BREAKFAST Time: _____ Meds/Insulin: _____						
Breakfast Total						
SNACK 1 Time: _____ Meds/Insulin: _____						
Snack 1 Total						
LUNCH Time: _____ Meds/Insulin: _____						
Lunch Total						
SNACK 2 Time: _____ Meds/Insulin: _____						
Snack 2 Total						
DINNER Time: _____ Meds/Insulin: _____						
Dinner Total						
Total Nutrition for the Day						

Water Consumption ⊔ ⊔ ⊔ ⊔ ⊔ ⊔ ⊔ ⊔ ⊔ ⊔   _____

EXERCISE & ACTIVITY LOG

	Time/Duration	Intensity/Calories

BLOOD SUGAR LOG

	Blood Sugar Level	
	Before	**After**
WAKING UP Time: _____	Sleep Hrs: _____ Fast. Hrs: _____	
BREAKFAST		
SNACK 1		
LUNCH		
SNACK 2		
DINNER		
BEDTIME	Go to Sleep Time: _____	

BLOOD PRESSURE & WEIGHT

Time	SYS/DIA	Pulse

WEIGHT: _____

NOTES/SCHEDULE

7 am	
8 am	
9 am	
10 am	
11 am	
12 am	
1 pm	
2 pm	
3 pm	
4 pm	
5 pm	
6 pm	
7 pm	
8 pm	

DATE: _____ SU | MO | TU | WE | TH | FR | SA   **Month/Week:** _____

FOOD, NUTRITION & MEDS

	Carbs	Sugar	Fiber	Protein	Fat	Calories
BREAKFAST Time: _____ Meds/Insulin: _____						
Breakfast Total						
SNACK 1 Time: _____ Meds/Insulin: _____						
Snack 1 Total						
LUNCH Time: _____ Meds/Insulin: _____						
Lunch Total						
SNACK 2 Time: _____ Meds/Insulin: _____						
Snack 2 Total						
DINNER Time: _____ Meds/Insulin: _____						
Dinner Total						
Total Nutrition for the Day						

Water Consumption ⊔ ⊔ ⊔ ⊔ ⊔ ⊔ ⊔ ⊔ ⊔ ⊔ _____

EXERCISE & ACTIVITY LOG

	Time/Duration	Intensity/Calories

BLOOD SUGAR LOG

	Blood Sugar Level	
	Before	**After**
WAKING UP Time: _____	Sleep Hrs: _____ Fast. Hrs: _____	
BREAKFAST		
SNACK 1		
LUNCH		
SNACK 2		
DINNER		
BEDTIME	Go to Sleep Time: _____	

BLOOD PRESSURE & WEIGHT

Time	SYS/DIA	Pulse

WEIGHT: _____

NOTES/SCHEDULE

7 am	
8 am	
9 am	
10 am	
11 am	
12 am	
1 pm	
2 pm	
3 pm	
4 pm	
5 pm	
6 pm	
7 pm	
8 pm	

DATE: _____ SU | MO | TU | WE | TH | FR | SA   **Month/Week:** _____

FOOD, NUTRITION & MEDS

	Carbs	Sugar	Fiber	Protein	Fat	Calories
BREAKFAST Time: _____ Meds/Insulin: _____						
Breakfast Total						
SNACK 1 Time: _____ Meds/Insulin: _____						
Snack 1 Total						
LUNCH Time: _____ Meds/Insulin: _____						
Lunch Total						
SNACK 2 Time: _____ Meds/Insulin: _____						
Snack 2 Total						
DINNER Time: _____ Meds/Insulin: _____						
Dinner Total						
Total Nutrition for the Day						

Water Consumption 🥛🥛🥛🥛🥛🥛🥛🥛🥛🥛 _____

BLOOD SUGAR LOG

	Blood Sugar Level	
	Before	**After**
WAKING UP Time: _____	Sleep Hrs: _____ Fast. Hrs: _____	
BREAKFAST		
SNACK 1		
LUNCH		
SNACK 2		
DINNER		
BEDTIME	Go to Sleep Time: _____	

BLOOD PRESSURE & WEIGHT

Time	SYS/DIA	Pulse
WEIGHT: _____		

NOTES/SCHEDULE

7 am	
8 am	
9 am	
10 am	
11 am	
12 am	
1 pm	
2 pm	
3 pm	
4 pm	
5 pm	
6 pm	
7 pm	
8 pm	

EXERCISE & ACTIVITY LOG

	Time/Duration	Intensity/Calories

DATE: _____   SU | MO | TU | WE | TH | FR | SA   **Month/Week:** _____

FOOD, NUTRITION & MEDS

		Carbs	Sugar	Fiber	Protein	Fat	Calories
BREAKFAST	Time: _____ Meds/Insulin: _____						
	Breakfast Total						
SNACK 1	Time: _____ Meds/Insulin: _____						
	Snack 1 Total						
LUNCH	Time: _____ Meds/Insulin: _____						
	Lunch Total						
SNACK 2	Time: _____ Meds/Insulin: _____						
	Snack 2 Total						
DINNER	Time: _____ Meds/Insulin: _____						
	Dinner Total						
	Total Nutrition for the Day						

Water Consumption   ⬜⬜⬜⬜⬜⬜⬜⬜⬜   _____

EXERCISE & ACTIVITY LOG

	Time/Duration	Intensity/Calories

BLOOD SUGAR LOG

	Blood Sugar Level	
	Before	**After**
WAKING UP Time: _____	Sleep Hrs: _____ Fast. Hrs: _____	
BREAKFAST		
SNACK 1		
LUNCH		
SNACK 2		
DINNER		
BEDTIME	Go to Sleep Time: _____	

BLOOD PRESSURE & WEIGHT

Time	SYS/DIA	Pulse
WEIGHT: _____		

NOTES/SCHEDULE

7 am	
8 am	
9 am	
10 am	
11 am	
12 am	
1 pm	
2 pm	
3 pm	
4 pm	
5 pm	
6 pm	
7 pm	
8 pm	

DATE: _____ SU | MO | TU | WE | TH | FR | SA   **Month/Week:** _____

FOOD, NUTRITION & MEDS

	Carbs	Sugar	Fiber	Protein	Fat	Calories
BREAKFAST Time: _____ Meds/Insulin: _____						
Breakfast Total						
SNACK 1 Time: _____ Meds/Insulin: _____						
Snack 1 Total						
LUNCH Time: _____ Meds/Insulin: _____						
Lunch Total						
SNACK 2 Time: _____ Meds/Insulin: _____						
Snack 2 Total						
DINNER Time: _____ Meds/Insulin: _____						
Dinner Total						
Total Nutrition for the Day						

Water Consumption ☐ ☐ ☐ ☐ ☐ ☐ ☐ ☐ ☐ _____

EXERCISE & ACTIVITY LOG

	Time/Duration	Intensity/Calories

BLOOD SUGAR LOG

	Blood Sugar Level	
	Before	**After**
WAKING UP Time: _____	Sleep Hrs: _____ Fast. Hrs: _____	
BREAKFAST		
SNACK 1		
LUNCH		
SNACK 2		
DINNER		
BEDTIME	Go to Sleep Time: _____	

BLOOD PRESSURE & WEIGHT

Time	SYS/DIA	Pulse

WEIGHT: _____

NOTES/SCHEDULE

7 am	
8 am	
9 am	
10 am	
11 am	
12 am	
1 pm	
2 pm	
3 pm	
4 pm	
5 pm	
6 pm	
7 pm	
8 pm	

DATE: _____   SU | MO | TU | WE | TH | FR | SA   **Month/Week:** _____

FOOD, NUTRITION & MEDS

	Carbs	Sugar	Fiber	Protein	Fat	Calories
BREAKFAST Time: _____ Meds/Insulin: _____						
Breakfast Total						
SNACK 1 Time: _____ Meds/Insulin: _____						
Snack 1 Total						
LUNCH Time: _____ Meds/Insulin: _____						
Lunch Total						
SNACK 2 Time: _____ Meds/Insulin: _____						
Snack 2 Total						
DINNER Time: _____ Meds/Insulin: _____						
Dinner Total						
Total Nutrition for the Day						

Water Consumption ☐ ☐ ☐ ☐ ☐ ☐ ☐ ☐ ☐ ☐   _____

EXERCISE & ACTIVITY LOG

	Time/Duration	Intensity/Calories

BLOOD SUGAR LOG

	Blood Sugar Level	
	Before	**After**
WAKING UP Time: _____	Sleep Hrs: _____ Fast. Hrs: _____	
BREAKFAST		
SNACK 1		
LUNCH		
SNACK 2		
DINNER		
BEDTIME	Go to Sleep Time: _____	

BLOOD PRESSURE & WEIGHT

Time	SYS/DIA	Pulse
WEIGHT: _____		

NOTES/SCHEDULE

7 am	
8 am	
9 am	
10 am	
11 am	
12 am	
1 pm	
2 pm	
3 pm	
4 pm	
5 pm	
6 pm	
7 pm	
8 pm	

DATE: _____   SU | MO | TU | WE | TH | FR | SA   **Month/Week:** _____

FOOD, NUTRITION & MEDS

	Carbs	Sugar	Fiber	Protein	Fat	Calories
BREAKFAST Time: _____ Meds/Insulin: _____						
Breakfast Total						
SNACK 1 Time: _____ Meds/Insulin: _____						
Snack 1 Total						
LUNCH Time: _____ Meds/Insulin: _____						
Lunch Total						
SNACK 2 Time: _____ Meds/Insulin: _____						
Snack 2 Total						
DINNER Time: _____ Meds/Insulin: _____						
Dinner Total						
Total Nutrition for the Day						

Water Consumption ▯ ▯ ▯ ▯ ▯ ▯ ▯ ▯ ▯ ▯ _____

EXERCISE & ACTIVITY LOG

	Time/Duration	Intensity/Calories

BLOOD SUGAR LOG

	Blood Sugar Level	
	Before	**After**
WAKING UP Time: _____	Sleep Hrs: _____ Fast. Hrs: _____	
BREAKFAST		
SNACK 1		
LUNCH		
SNACK 2		
DINNER		
BEDTIME	Go to Sleep Time: _____	

BLOOD PRESSURE & WEIGHT

Time	SYS/DIA	Pulse
WEIGHT: _____		

NOTES/SCHEDULE

7 am	
8 am	
9 am	
10 am	
11 am	
12 am	
1 pm	
2 pm	
3 pm	
4 pm	
5 pm	
6 pm	
7 pm	
8 pm	

DATE: _____   SU | MO | TU | WE | TH | FR | SA   **Month/Week:** _____

FOOD, NUTRITION & MEDS

	Carbs	Sugar	Fiber	Protein	Fat	Calories
BREAKFAST Time: _____ Meds/Insulin: _____						
Breakfast Total						
SNACK 1 Time: _____ Meds/Insulin: _____						
Snack 1 Total						
LUNCH Time: _____ Meds/Insulin: _____						
Lunch Total						
SNACK 2 Time: _____ Meds/Insulin: _____						
Snack 2 Total						
DINNER Time: _____ Meds/Insulin: _____						
Dinner Total						
Total Nutrition for the Day						

Water Consumption ⊔ ⊔ ⊔ ⊔ ⊔ ⊔ ⊔ ⊔ ⊔ ⊔ _____

BLOOD SUGAR LOG

	Blood Sugar Level	
	Before	**After**
WAKING UP Time: _____	Sleep Hrs: _____ Fast. Hrs: _____	
BREAKFAST		
SNACK 1		
LUNCH		
SNACK 2		
DINNER		
BEDTIME	Go to Sleep Time: _____	

BLOOD PRESSURE & WEIGHT

Time	SYS/DIA	Pulse

WEIGHT: _____

NOTES/SCHEDULE

7 am	
8 am	
9 am	
10 am	
11 am	
12 am	
1 pm	
2 pm	
3 pm	
4 pm	
5 pm	
6 pm	
7 pm	
8 pm	

EXERCISE & ACTIVITY LOG

	Time/Duration	Intensity/Calories

DATE: _____ SU | MO | TU | WE | TH | FR | SA   **Month/Week:** _____

FOOD, NUTRITION & MEDS

	Carbs	Sugar	Fiber	Protein	Fat	Calories
BREAKFAST Time: _____ Meds/Insulin: _____						
Breakfast Total						
SNACK 1 Time: _____ Meds/Insulin: _____						
Snack 1 Total						
LUNCH Time: _____ Meds/Insulin: _____						
Lunch Total						
SNACK 2 Time: _____ Meds/Insulin: _____						
Snack 2 Total						
DINNER Time: _____ Meds/Insulin: _____						
Dinner Total						
Total Nutrition for the Day						

Water Consumption ☐ ☐ ☐ ☐ ☐ ☐ ☐ ☐ ☐ _____

EXERCISE & ACTIVITY LOG

	Time/Duration	Intensity/Calories

BLOOD SUGAR LOG

	Blood Sugar Level	
	Before	**After**
WAKING UP Time: _____	Sleep Hrs: _____ Fast. Hrs: _____	
BREAKFAST		
SNACK 1		
LUNCH		
SNACK 2		
DINNER		
BEDTIME	Go to Sleep Time: _____	

BLOOD PRESSURE & WEIGHT

Time	SYS/DIA	Pulse

WEIGHT: _____

NOTES/SCHEDULE

7 am	
8 am	
9 am	
10 am	
11 am	
12 am	
1 pm	
2 pm	
3 pm	
4 pm	
5 pm	
6 pm	
7 pm	
8 pm	

DATE: _____ SU | MO | TU | WE | TH | FR | SA   **Month/Week:** _____

FOOD, NUTRITION & MEDS

	Carbs	Sugar	Fiber	Protein	Fat	Calories

BREAKFAST Time: _____ Meds/Insulin: _____

Breakfast Total						

SNACK 1 Time: _____ Meds/Insulin: _____

Snack 1 Total						

LUNCH Time: _____ Meds/Insulin: _____

Lunch Total						

SNACK 2 Time: _____ Meds/Insulin: _____

Snack 2 Total						

DINNER Time: _____ Meds/Insulin: _____

Dinner Total						
Total Nutrition for the Day						

Water Consumption ⬜⬜⬜⬜⬜⬜⬜⬜⬜⬜ _____

EXERCISE & ACTIVITY LOG

	Time/Duration	Intensity/Calories

BLOOD SUGAR LOG

	Blood Sugar Level	
	Before	**After**
WAKING UP Time: _____	Sleep Hrs: _____ Fast. Hrs: _____	
BREAKFAST		
SNACK 1		
LUNCH		
SNACK 2		
DINNER		
BEDTIME	Go to Sleep Time: _____	

BLOOD PRESSURE & WEIGHT

Time	SYS/DIA	Pulse
WEIGHT: _____		

NOTES/SCHEDULE

7 am	
8 am	
9 am	
10 am	
11 am	
12 am	
1 pm	
2 pm	
3 pm	
4 pm	
5 pm	
6 pm	
7 pm	
8 pm	

DATE: _____   SU | MO | TU | WE | TH | FR | SA

Month/Week: _____

FOOD, NUTRITION & MEDS

	Carbs	Sugar	Fiber	Protein	Fat	Calories
BREAKFAST Time: _____ Meds/Insulin: _____						
Breakfast Total						
SNACK 1 Time: _____ Meds/Insulin: _____						
Snack 1 Total						
LUNCH Time: _____ Meds/Insulin: _____						
Lunch Total						
SNACK 2 Time: _____ Meds/Insulin: _____						
Snack 2 Total						
DINNER Time: _____ Meds/Insulin: _____						
Dinner Total						
Total Nutrition for the Day						

Water Consumption ⬜ ⬜ ⬜ ⬜ ⬜ ⬜ ⬜ ⬜ ⬜ ⬜   _____

BLOOD SUGAR LOG

	Blood Sugar Level	
	Before	**After**
WAKING UP Time: _____	Sleep Hrs: _____ Fast. Hrs: _____	
BREAKFAST		
SNACK 1		
LUNCH		
SNACK 2		
DINNER		
BEDTIME	Go to Sleep Time: _____	

BLOOD PRESSURE & WEIGHT

Time	SYS/DIA	Pulse

WEIGHT: _____

NOTES/SCHEDULE

7 am	
8 am	
9 am	
10 am	
11 am	
12 am	
1 pm	
2 pm	
3 pm	
4 pm	
5 pm	
6 pm	
7 pm	
8 pm	

EXERCISE & ACTIVITY LOG

	Time/Duration	Intensity/Calories

DATE: _____ SU | MO | TU | WE | TH | FR | SA   **Month/Week:** _____

FOOD, NUTRITION & MEDS

	Carbs	Sugar	Fiber	Protein	Fat	Calories
BREAKFAST Time: _____ Meds/Insulin: _____						
Breakfast Total						
SNACK 1 Time: _____ Meds/Insulin: _____						
Snack 1 Total						
LUNCH Time: _____ Meds/Insulin: _____						
Lunch Total						
SNACK 2 Time: _____ Meds/Insulin: _____						
Snack 2 Total						
DINNER Time: _____ Meds/Insulin: _____						
Dinner Total						
Total Nutrition for the Day						

Water Consumption ⬚⬚⬚⬚⬚⬚⬚⬚⬚⬚ _____

BLOOD SUGAR LOG

	Blood Sugar Level	
	Before	**After**
WAKING UP Time: _____	Sleep Hrs: _____ Fast. Hrs: _____	
BREAKFAST		
SNACK 1		
LUNCH		
SNACK 2		
DINNER		
BEDTIME	Go to Sleep Time: _____	

BLOOD PRESSURE & WEIGHT

Time	SYS/DIA	Pulse

WEIGHT: _____

NOTES/SCHEDULE

7 am	
8 am	
9 am	
10 am	
11 am	
12 am	
1 pm	
2 pm	
3 pm	
4 pm	
5 pm	
6 pm	
7 pm	
8 pm	

EXERCISE & ACTIVITY LOG

	Time/Duration	Intensity/Calories

DATE: _____ SU | MO | TU | WE | TH | FR | SA   **Month/Week:** _____

FOOD, NUTRITION & MEDS

	Carbs	Sugar	Fiber	Protein	Fat	Calories
BREAKFAST Time: _____ Meds/Insulin: _____						
Breakfast Total						
SNACK 1 Time: _____ Meds/Insulin: _____						
Snack 1 Total						
LUNCH Time: _____ Meds/Insulin: _____						
Lunch Total						
SNACK 2 Time: _____ Meds/Insulin: _____						
Snack 2 Total						
DINNER Time: _____ Meds/Insulin: _____						
Dinner Total						
Total Nutrition for the Day						

Water Consumption 🥛🥛🥛🥛🥛🥛🥛🥛🥛🥛 _____

BLOOD SUGAR LOG

	Blood Sugar Level	
	Before	**After**
WAKING UP Time: _____	Sleep Hrs: _____ Fast. Hrs: _____	
BREAKFAST		
SNACK 1		
LUNCH		
SNACK 2		
DINNER		
BEDTIME	Go to Sleep Time: _____	

BLOOD PRESSURE & WEIGHT

Time	SYS/DIA	Pulse

WEIGHT: _____

NOTES/SCHEDULE

7 am	
8 am	
9 am	
10 am	
11 am	
12 am	
1 pm	
2 pm	
3 pm	
4 pm	
5 pm	
6 pm	
7 pm	
8 pm	

EXERCISE & ACTIVITY LOG

	Time/Duration	Intensity/Calories

DATE: _____ SU | MO | TU | WE | TH | FR | SA   **Month/Week:** _____

FOOD, NUTRITION & MEDS

	Carbs	Sugar	Fiber	Protein	Fat	Calories
BREAKFAST Time: _____ Meds/Insulin: _____						
Breakfast Total						
SNACK 1 Time: _____ Meds/Insulin: _____						
Snack 1 Total						
LUNCH Time: _____ Meds/Insulin: _____						
Lunch Total						
SNACK 2 Time: _____ Meds/Insulin: _____						
Snack 2 Total						
DINNER Time: _____ Meds/Insulin: _____						
Dinner Total						
Total Nutrition for the Day						

Water Consumption ⌷ ⌷ ⌷ ⌷ ⌷ ⌷ ⌷ ⌷ ⌷ ⌷ _____

BLOOD SUGAR LOG

	Blood Sugar Level	
	Before	**After**
WAKING UP Time: _____	Sleep Hrs: _____ Fast. Hrs: _____	
BREAKFAST		
SNACK 1		
LUNCH		
SNACK 2		
DINNER		
BEDTIME	Go to Sleep Time: _____	

BLOOD PRESSURE & WEIGHT

Time	SYS/DIA	Pulse

WEIGHT: _____

NOTES/SCHEDULE

7 am	
8 am	
9 am	
10 am	
11 am	
12 am	
1 pm	
2 pm	
3 pm	
4 pm	
5 pm	
6 pm	
7 pm	
8 pm	

EXERCISE & ACTIVITY LOG

	Time/Duration	Intensity/Calories

DATE: ---------------------- SU | MO | TU | WE | TH | FR | SA   **Month/Week:** ----------------------

FOOD, NUTRITION & MEDS

	Carbs	Sugar	Fiber	Protein	Fat	Calories
BREAKFAST Time: ------------- Meds/Insulin: -------------------------						
Breakfast Total						
SNACK 1 Time: ------------- Meds/Insulin: -------------------------						
Snack 1 Total						
LUNCH Time: ------------- Meds/Insulin: -------------------------						
Lunch Total						
SNACK 2 Time: ------------- Meds/Insulin: -------------------------						
Snack 2 Total						
DINNER Time: ------------- Meds/Insulin: -------------------------						
Dinner Total						
Total Nutrition for the Day						

Water Consumption ⛆ ⛆ ⛆ ⛆ ⛆ ⛆ ⛆ ⛆ ⛆ ⛆ -------------

EXERCISE & ACTIVITY LOG

	Time/Duration	Intensity/Calories

BLOOD SUGAR LOG

	Blood Sugar Level	
	Before	**After**
WAKING UP Time: ---------	Sleep Hrs: ------------ Fast. Hrs: ------------	
BREAKFAST		
SNACK 1		
LUNCH		
SNACK 2		
DINNER		
BEDTIME	Go to Sleep Time: ------------	

BLOOD PRESSURE & WEIGHT

Time	SYS/DIA	Pulse

WEIGHT: --------------------

NOTES/SCHEDULE

7 am	
8 am	
9 am	
10 am	
11 am	
12 am	
1 pm	
2 pm	
3 pm	
4 pm	
5 pm	
6 pm	
7 pm	
8 pm	

DATE: _____ SU | MO | TU | WE | TH | FR | SA

Month/Week: _____

FOOD, NUTRITION & MEDS

	Carbs	Sugar	Fiber	Protein	Fat	Calories
BREAKFAST Time: _____ Meds/Insulin: _____						
Breakfast Total						
SNACK 1 Time: _____ Meds/Insulin: _____						
Snack 1 Total						
LUNCH Time: _____ Meds/Insulin: _____						
Lunch Total						
SNACK 2 Time: _____ Meds/Insulin: _____						
Snack 2 Total						
DINNER Time: _____ Meds/Insulin: _____						
Dinner Total						
Total Nutrition for the Day						

Water Consumption ⛆ ⛆ ⛆ ⛆ ⛆ ⛆ ⛆ ⛆ ⛆ ⛆ _____

EXERCISE & ACTIVITY LOG

	Time/Duration	Intensity/Calories

BLOOD SUGAR LOG

	Blood Sugar Level	
	Before	**After**
WAKING UP Time: _____	Sleep Hrs: _____ Fast. Hrs: _____	
BREAKFAST		
SNACK 1		
LUNCH		
SNACK 2		
DINNER		
BEDTIME	Go to Sleep Time: _____	

BLOOD PRESSURE & WEIGHT

Time	SYS/DIA	Pulse

WEIGHT: _____

NOTES/SCHEDULE

7 am	
8 am	
9 am	
10 am	
11 am	
12 am	
1 pm	
2 pm	
3 pm	
4 pm	
5 pm	
6 pm	
7 pm	
8 pm	

DATE: _____ SU | MO | TU | WE | TH | FR | SA   **Month/Week:** _____

FOOD, NUTRITION & MEDS

	Carbs	Sugar	Fiber	Protein	Fat	Calories
BREAKFAST Time: _____ Meds/Insulin: _____						
Breakfast Total						
SNACK 1 Time: _____ Meds/Insulin: _____						
Snack 1 Total						
LUNCH Time: _____ Meds/Insulin: _____						
Lunch Total						
SNACK 2 Time: _____ Meds/Insulin: _____						
Snack 2 Total						
DINNER Time: _____ Meds/Insulin: _____						
Dinner Total						
Total Nutrition for the Day						

Water Consumption ▯ ▯ ▯ ▯ ▯ ▯ ▯ ▯ ▯ ▯ _____

EXERCISE & ACTIVITY LOG

	Time/Duration	Intensity/Calories

BLOOD SUGAR LOG

	Blood Sugar Level	
	Before	**After**
WAKING UP Time: _____	Sleep Hrs: _____ Fast. Hrs: _____	
BREAKFAST		
SNACK 1		
LUNCH		
SNACK 2		
DINNER		
BEDTIME	Go to Sleep Time: _____	

BLOOD PRESSURE & WEIGHT

Time	SYS/DIA	Pulse

WEIGHT: _____

NOTES/SCHEDULE

7 am	
8 am	
9 am	
10 am	
11 am	
12 am	
1 pm	
2 pm	
3 pm	
4 pm	
5 pm	
6 pm	
7 pm	
8 pm	

DATE: _____   SU | MO | TU | WE | TH | FR | SA   **Month/Week:** _____

FOOD, NUTRITION & MEDS

	Carbs	Sugar	Fiber	Protein	Fat	Calories
BREAKFAST Time: _____ Meds/Insulin: _____						
Breakfast Total						
SNACK 1 Time: _____ Meds/Insulin: _____						
Snack 1 Total						
LUNCH Time: _____ Meds/Insulin: _____						
Lunch Total						
SNACK 2 Time: _____ Meds/Insulin: _____						
Snack 2 Total						
DINNER Time: _____ Meds/Insulin: _____						
Dinner Total						
Total Nutrition for the Day						

Water Consumption ☐ ☐ ☐ ☐ ☐ ☐ ☐ ☐ ☐ ☐ _____

BLOOD SUGAR LOG

	Blood Sugar Level	
	Before	After
WAKING UP Time: _____	Sleep Hrs: _____ Fast. Hrs: _____	
BREAKFAST		
SNACK 1		
LUNCH		
SNACK 2		
DINNER		
BEDTIME	Go to Sleep Time: _____	

BLOOD PRESSURE & WEIGHT

Time	SYS/DIA	Pulse
WEIGHT: _____		

NOTES/SCHEDULE

7 am	
8 am	
9 am	
10 am	
11 am	
12 am	
1 pm	
2 pm	
3 pm	
4 pm	
5 pm	
6 pm	
7 pm	
8 pm	

EXERCISE & ACTIVITY LOG

	Time/Duration	Intensity/Calories

DATE: _____ SU | MO | TU | WE | TH | FR | SA

Month/Week: _____

FOOD, NUTRITION & MEDS

	Carbs	Sugar	Fiber	Protein	Fat	Calories
BREAKFAST Time: _____ Meds/Insulin: _____						
Breakfast Total						
SNACK 1 Time: _____ Meds/Insulin: _____						
Snack 1 Total						
LUNCH Time: _____ Meds/Insulin: _____						
Lunch Total						
SNACK 2 Time: _____ Meds/Insulin: _____						
Snack 2 Total						
DINNER Time: _____ Meds/Insulin: _____						
Dinner Total						
Total Nutrition for the Day						

Water Consumption 🥛🥛🥛🥛🥛🥛🥛🥛🥛🥛 _____

EXERCISE & ACTIVITY LOG

	Time/Duration	Intensity/Calories

BLOOD SUGAR LOG

	Blood Sugar Level	
	Before	**After**
WAKING UP Time: _____	Sleep Hrs: _____ Fast. Hrs: _____	
BREAKFAST		
SNACK 1		
LUNCH		
SNACK 2		
DINNER		
BEDTIME	Go to Sleep Time: _____	

BLOOD PRESSURE & WEIGHT

Time	SYS/DIA	Pulse
WEIGHT: _____		

NOTES/SCHEDULE

7 am	
8 am	
9 am	
10 am	
11 am	
12 am	
1 pm	
2 pm	
3 pm	
4 pm	
5 pm	
6 pm	
7 pm	
8 pm	

DATE: _____ SU | MO | TU | WE | TH | FR | SA   **Month/Week:** _____

FOOD, NUTRITION & MEDS

	Carbs	Sugar	Fiber	Protein	Fat	Calories
BREAKFAST Time: _____ Meds/Insulin: _____						
Breakfast Total						
SNACK 1 Time: _____ Meds/Insulin: _____						
Snack 1 Total						
LUNCH Time: _____ Meds/Insulin: _____						
Lunch Total						
SNACK 2 Time: _____ Meds/Insulin: _____						
Snack 2 Total						
DINNER Time: _____ Meds/Insulin: _____						
Dinner Total						
Total Nutrition for the Day						

Water Consumption ▢ ▢ ▢ ▢ ▢ ▢ ▢ ▢ ▢ ▢ _____

EXERCISE & ACTIVITY LOG

	Time/Duration	Intensity/Calories

BLOOD SUGAR LOG

	Blood Sugar Level	
	Before	**After**
WAKING UP Time: _____	Sleep Hrs: _____ Fast. Hrs: _____	
BREAKFAST		
SNACK 1		
LUNCH		
SNACK 2		
DINNER		
BEDTIME	Go to Sleep Time: _____	

BLOOD PRESSURE & WEIGHT

Time	SYS/DIA	Pulse

WEIGHT: _____

NOTES/SCHEDULE

7 am	
8 am	
9 am	
10 am	
11 am	
12 am	
1 pm	
2 pm	
3 pm	
4 pm	
5 pm	
6 pm	
7 pm	
8 pm	

DATE: _____ SU | MO | TU | WE | TH | FR | SA   **Month/Week:** _____

FOOD, NUTRITION & MEDS

	Carbs	Sugar	Fiber	Protein	Fat	Calories
BREAKFAST Time: _____ Meds/Insulin: _____						
Breakfast Total						
SNACK 1 Time: _____ Meds/Insulin: _____						
Snack 1 Total						
LUNCH Time: _____ Meds/Insulin: _____						
Lunch Total						
SNACK 2 Time: _____ Meds/Insulin: _____						
Snack 2 Total						
DINNER Time: _____ Meds/Insulin: _____						
Dinner Total						
Total Nutrition for the Day						

Water Consumption ⎕ ⎕ ⎕ ⎕ ⎕ ⎕ ⎕ ⎕ ⎕ ⎕ _____

BLOOD SUGAR LOG

	Blood Sugar Level	
	Before	**After**
WAKING UP Time: _____	Sleep Hrs: _____ Fast. Hrs: _____	
BREAKFAST		
SNACK 1		
LUNCH		
SNACK 2		
DINNER		
BEDTIME	Go to Sleep Time: _____	

BLOOD PRESSURE & WEIGHT

Time	SYS/DIA	Pulse

WEIGHT: _____

NOTES/SCHEDULE

7 am	
8 am	
9 am	
10 am	
11 am	
12 am	
1 pm	
2 pm	
3 pm	
4 pm	
5 pm	
6 pm	
7 pm	
8 pm	

EXERCISE & ACTIVITY LOG

	Time/Duration	Intensity/Calories

DATE: _____   SU | MO | TU | WE | TH | FR | SA   **Month/Week:** _____

FOOD, NUTRITION & MEDS

	Carbs	Sugar	Fiber	Protein	Fat	Calories
BREAKFAST Time: _____ Meds/Insulin: _____						
Breakfast Total						
SNACK 1 Time: _____ Meds/Insulin: _____						
Snack 1 Total						
LUNCH Time: _____ Meds/Insulin: _____						
Lunch Total						
SNACK 2 Time: _____ Meds/Insulin: _____						
Snack 2 Total						
DINNER Time: _____ Meds/Insulin: _____						
Dinner Total						
Total Nutrition for the Day						

Water Consumption 🥛🥛🥛🥛🥛🥛🥛🥛🥛 _____

BLOOD SUGAR LOG

	Blood Sugar Level	
	Before	**After**
WAKING UP Time: _____ Sleep Hrs: _____ Fast. Hrs: _____		
BREAKFAST		
SNACK 1		
LUNCH		
SNACK 2		
DINNER		
BEDTIME Go to Sleep Time: _____		

BLOOD PRESSURE & WEIGHT

Time	SYS/DIA	Pulse

WEIGHT: _____

NOTES/SCHEDULE

7 am	
8 am	
9 am	
10 am	
11 am	
12 am	
1 pm	
2 pm	
3 pm	
4 pm	
5 pm	
6 pm	
7 pm	
8 pm	

EXERCISE & ACTIVITY LOG

	Time/Duration	Intensity/Calories

DATE: _____ SU | MO | TU | WE | TH | FR | SA   **Month/Week:** _____

FOOD, NUTRITION & MEDS

	Carbs	Sugar	Fiber	Protein	Fat	Calories
BREAKFAST Time: _____ Meds/Insulin: _____						
Breakfast Total						
SNACK 1 Time: _____ Meds/Insulin: _____						
Snack 1 Total						
LUNCH Time: _____ Meds/Insulin: _____						
Lunch Total						
SNACK 2 Time: _____ Meds/Insulin: _____						
Snack 2 Total						
DINNER Time: _____ Meds/Insulin: _____						
Dinner Total						
Total Nutrition for the Day						

Water Consumption ▯ ▯ ▯ ▯ ▯ ▯ ▯ ▯ ▯ ▯ _____

EXERCISE & ACTIVITY LOG

	Time/Duration	Intensity/Calories

BLOOD SUGAR LOG

	Blood Sugar Level	
	Before	**After**
WAKING UP Time: _____	Sleep Hrs: _____ Fast. Hrs: _____	
BREAKFAST		
SNACK 1		
LUNCH		
SNACK 2		
DINNER		
BEDTIME	Go to Sleep Time: _____	

BLOOD PRESSURE & WEIGHT

Time	SYS/DIA	Pulse

WEIGHT: _____

NOTES/SCHEDULE

7 am	
8 am	
9 am	
10 am	
11 am	
12 am	
1 pm	
2 pm	
3 pm	
4 pm	
5 pm	
6 pm	
7 pm	
8 pm	

DATE: _____ SU | MO | TU | WE | TH | FR | SA

Month/Week: _____

FOOD, NUTRITION & MEDS

	Carbs	Sugar	Fiber	Protein	Fat	Calories
BREAKFAST Time: _____ Meds/Insulin: _____						
Breakfast Total						
SNACK 1 Time: _____ Meds/Insulin: _____						
Snack 1 Total						
LUNCH Time: _____ Meds/Insulin: _____						
Lunch Total						
SNACK 2 Time: _____ Meds/Insulin: _____						
Snack 2 Total						
DINNER Time: _____ Meds/Insulin: _____						
Dinner Total						
Total Nutrition for the Day						

Water Consumption ⬜⬜⬜⬜⬜⬜⬜⬜⬜⬜ _____

BLOOD SUGAR LOG

	Blood Sugar Level	
	Before	**After**
WAKING UP Time: _____	Sleep Hrs: _____ Fast. Hrs: _____	
BREAKFAST		
SNACK 1		
LUNCH		
SNACK 2		
DINNER		
BEDTIME	Go to Sleep Time: _____	

BLOOD PRESSURE & WEIGHT

Time	SYS/DIA	Pulse

WEIGHT: _____

NOTES/SCHEDULE

7 am	
8 am	
9 am	
10 am	
11 am	
12 am	
1 pm	
2 pm	
3 pm	
4 pm	
5 pm	
6 pm	
7 pm	
8 pm	

EXERCISE & ACTIVITY LOG

	Time/Duration	Intensity/Calories

DATE: _____ SU | MO | TU | WE | TH | FR | SA

Month/Week: _____

FOOD, NUTRITION & MEDS

	Carbs	Sugar	Fiber	Protein	Fat	Calories
BREAKFAST Time: _____ Meds/Insulin: _____						
Breakfast Total						
SNACK 1 Time: _____ Meds/Insulin: _____						
Snack 1 Total						
LUNCH Time: _____ Meds/Insulin: _____						
Lunch Total						
SNACK 2 Time: _____ Meds/Insulin: _____						
Snack 2 Total						
DINNER Time: _____ Meds/Insulin: _____						
Dinner Total						
Total Nutrition for the Day						

Water Consumption ⬜⬜⬜⬜⬜⬜⬜⬜⬜⬜ _____

EXERCISE & ACTIVITY LOG

	Time/Duration	Intensity/Calories

BLOOD SUGAR LOG

	Blood Sugar Level	
	Before	**After**
WAKING UP Time: _____	Sleep Hrs: _____ Fast. Hrs: _____	
BREAKFAST		
SNACK 1		
LUNCH		
SNACK 2		
DINNER		
BEDTIME	Go to Sleep Time: _____	

BLOOD PRESSURE & WEIGHT

Time	SYS/DIA	Pulse

WEIGHT: _____

NOTES/SCHEDULE

7 am	
8 am	
9 am	
10 am	
11 am	
12 am	
1 pm	
2 pm	
3 pm	
4 pm	
5 pm	
6 pm	
7 pm	
8 pm	

DATE: _____   SU | MO | TU | WE | TH | FR | SA   **Month/Week:** _____

FOOD, NUTRITION & MEDS

	Carbs	Sugar	Fiber	Protein	Fat	Calories
BREAKFAST Time: _____ Meds/Insulin: _____						
Breakfast Total						
SNACK 1 Time: _____ Meds/Insulin: _____						
Snack 1 Total						
LUNCH Time: _____ Meds/Insulin: _____						
Lunch Total						
SNACK 2 Time: _____ Meds/Insulin: _____						
Snack 2 Total						
DINNER Time: _____ Meds/Insulin: _____						
Dinner Total						
Total Nutrition for the Day						

Water Consumption ☐ ☐ ☐ ☐ ☐ ☐ ☐ ☐ ☐   _____

BLOOD SUGAR LOG

	Blood Sugar Level	
	Before	**After**
WAKING UP Time: _____	Sleep Hrs: _____ Fast. Hrs: _____	
BREAKFAST		
SNACK 1		
LUNCH		
SNACK 2		
DINNER		
BEDTIME	Go to Sleep Time: _____	

BLOOD PRESSURE & WEIGHT

Time	**SYS/DIA**	**Pulse**

WEIGHT: _____

NOTES/SCHEDULE

7 am	
8 am	
9 am	
10 am	
11 am	
12 am	
1 pm	
2 pm	
3 pm	
4 pm	
5 pm	
6 pm	
7 pm	
8 pm	

EXERCISE & ACTIVITY LOG

	Time/Duration	**Intensity/Calories**

DATE: _____ SU | MO | TU | WE | TH | FR | SA **Month/Week:** _____

FOOD, NUTRITION & MEDS

	Carbs	Sugar	Fiber	Protein	Fat	Calories
BREAKFAST Time: _____ Meds/Insulin: _____						
Breakfast Total						
SNACK 1 Time: _____ Meds/Insulin: _____						
Snack 1 Total						
LUNCH Time: _____ Meds/Insulin: _____						
Lunch Total						
SNACK 2 Time: _____ Meds/Insulin: _____						
Snack 2 Total						
DINNER Time: _____ Meds/Insulin: _____						
Dinner Total						
Total Nutrition for the Day						

Water Consumption ⬚ ⬚ ⬚ ⬚ ⬚ ⬚ ⬚ ⬚ ⬚ ⬚ _____

BLOOD SUGAR LOG

	Blood Sugar Level	
	Before	**After**
WAKING UP Time: _____	Sleep Hrs: _____ Fast. Hrs: _____	
BREAKFAST		
SNACK 1		
LUNCH		
SNACK 2		
DINNER		
BEDTIME	Go to Sleep Time: _____	

BLOOD PRESSURE & WEIGHT

Time	SYS/DIA	Pulse

WEIGHT: _____

NOTES/SCHEDULE

7 am	
8 am	
9 am	
10 am	
11 am	
12 am	
1 pm	
2 pm	
3 pm	
4 pm	
5 pm	
6 pm	
7 pm	
8 pm	

EXERCISE & ACTIVITY LOG

	Time/Duration	Intensity/Calories

DATE: _____ SU | MO | TU | WE | TH | FR | SA   **Month/Week:** _____

FOOD, NUTRITION & MEDS

	Carbs	Sugar	Fiber	Protein	Fat	Calories
BREAKFAST Time: _____ Meds/Insulin: _____						
Breakfast Total						
SNACK 1 Time: _____ Meds/Insulin: _____						
Snack 1 Total						
LUNCH Time: _____ Meds/Insulin: _____						
Lunch Total						
SNACK 2 Time: _____ Meds/Insulin: _____						
Snack 2 Total						
DINNER Time: _____ Meds/Insulin: _____						
Dinner Total						
Total Nutrition for the Day						

Water Consumption ▯ ▯ ▯ ▯ ▯ ▯ ▯ ▯ ▯ ▯   _____

EXERCISE & ACTIVITY LOG

	Time/Duration	Intensity/Calories

BLOOD SUGAR LOG

	Blood Sugar Level	
	Before	**After**
WAKING UP Time: _____	Sleep Hrs: _____ Fast. Hrs: _____	
BREAKFAST		
SNACK 1		
LUNCH		
SNACK 2		
DINNER		
BEDTIME	Go to Sleep Time: _____	

BLOOD PRESSURE & WEIGHT

Time	SYS/DIA	Pulse

WEIGHT: _____

NOTES/SCHEDULE

7 am	
8 am	
9 am	
10 am	
11 am	
12 am	
1 pm	
2 pm	
3 pm	
4 pm	
5 pm	
6 pm	
7 pm	
8 pm	

DATE: _____ SU | MO | TU | WE | TH | FR | SA   **Month/Week:** _____

FOOD, NUTRITION & MEDS

	Carbs	Sugar	Fiber	Protein	Fat	Calories
BREAKFAST Time: _____ Meds/Insulin: _____						
Breakfast Total						
SNACK 1 Time: _____ Meds/Insulin: _____						
Snack 1 Total						
LUNCH Time: _____ Meds/Insulin: _____						
Lunch Total						
SNACK 2 Time: _____ Meds/Insulin: _____						
Snack 2 Total						
DINNER Time: _____ Meds/Insulin: _____						
Dinner Total						
Total Nutrition for the Day						

Water Consumption ⬜ ⬜ ⬜ ⬜ ⬜ ⬜ ⬜ ⬜ ⬜ ⬜ _____

EXERCISE & ACTIVITY LOG

	Time/Duration	Intensity/Calories

BLOOD SUGAR LOG

	Blood Sugar Level	
	Before	**After**
WAKING UP Time: _____	Sleep Hrs: _____ Fast. Hrs: _____	
BREAKFAST		
SNACK 1		
LUNCH		
SNACK 2		
DINNER		
BEDTIME	Go to Sleep Time: _____	

BLOOD PRESSURE & WEIGHT

Time	SYS/DIA	Pulse
WEIGHT: _____		

NOTES/SCHEDULE

7 am	
8 am	
9 am	
10 am	
11 am	
12 am	
1 pm	
2 pm	
3 pm	
4 pm	
5 pm	
6 pm	
7 pm	
8 pm	

DATE: _____ SU | MO | TU | WE | TH | FR | SA   **Month/Week:** _____

FOOD, NUTRITION & MEDS

	Carbs	Sugar	Fiber	Protein	Fat	Calories
BREAKFAST Time: _____ Meds/Insulin: _____						
Breakfast Total						
SNACK 1 Time: _____ Meds/Insulin: _____						
Snack 1 Total						
LUNCH Time: _____ Meds/Insulin: _____						
Lunch Total						
SNACK 2 Time: _____ Meds/Insulin: _____						
Snack 2 Total						
DINNER Time: _____ Meds/Insulin: _____						
Dinner Total						
Total Nutrition for the Day						

Water Consumption ⛾ ⛾ ⛾ ⛾ ⛾ ⛾ ⛾ ⛾ ⛾ ⛾ _____

EXERCISE & ACTIVITY LOG

	Time/Duration	Intensity/Calories

BLOOD SUGAR LOG

	Blood Sugar Level	
	Before	**After**
WAKING UP Time: _____	Sleep Hrs: _____ Fast. Hrs: _____	
BREAKFAST		
SNACK 1		
LUNCH		
SNACK 2		
DINNER		
BEDTIME	Go to Sleep Time: _____	

BLOOD PRESSURE & WEIGHT

Time	SYS/DIA	Pulse

WEIGHT: _____

NOTES/SCHEDULE

7 am	
8 am	
9 am	
10 am	
11 am	
12 am	
1 pm	
2 pm	
3 pm	
4 pm	
5 pm	
6 pm	
7 pm	
8 pm	

DATE: _____ SU | MO | TU | WE | TH | FR | SA   **Month/Week:** _____

FOOD, NUTRITION & MEDS

	Carbs	Sugar	Fiber	Protein	Fat	Calories
BREAKFAST Time: _____ Meds/Insulin: _____						
Breakfast Total						
SNACK 1 Time: _____ Meds/Insulin: _____						
Snack 1 Total						
LUNCH Time: _____ Meds/Insulin: _____						
Lunch Total						
SNACK 2 Time: _____ Meds/Insulin: _____						
Snack 2 Total						
DINNER Time: _____ Meds/Insulin: _____						
Dinner Total						
Total Nutrition for the Day						

Water Consumption ▢ ▢ ▢ ▢ ▢ ▢ ▢ ▢ ▢ ▢ _____

EXERCISE & ACTIVITY LOG

	Time/Duration	Intensity/Calories

BLOOD SUGAR LOG

	Blood Sugar Level	
	Before	**After**
WAKING UP Time: _____	Sleep Hrs: _____ Fast. Hrs: _____	
BREAKFAST		
SNACK 1		
LUNCH		
SNACK 2		
DINNER		
BEDTIME	Go to Sleep Time: _____	

BLOOD PRESSURE & WEIGHT

Time	SYS/DIA	Pulse
WEIGHT: _____		

NOTES/SCHEDULE

7 am	
8 am	
9 am	
10 am	
11 am	
12 am	
1 pm	
2 pm	
3 pm	
4 pm	
5 pm	
6 pm	
7 pm	
8 pm	

DATE: _____ SU | MO | TU | WE | TH | FR | SA   **Month/Week:** _____

FOOD, NUTRITION & MEDS

	Carbs	Sugar	Fiber	Protein	Fat	Calories
BREAKFAST Time: _____ Meds/Insulin: _____						
Breakfast Total						
SNACK 1 Time: _____ Meds/Insulin: _____						
Snack 1 Total						
LUNCH Time: _____ Meds/Insulin: _____						
Lunch Total						
SNACK 2 Time: _____ Meds/Insulin: _____						
Snack 2 Total						
DINNER Time: _____ Meds/Insulin: _____						
Dinner Total						
Total Nutrition for the Day						

Water Consumption 🥛🥛🥛🥛🥛🥛🥛🥛🥛🥛 _____

EXERCISE & ACTIVITY LOG

	Time/Duration	Intensity/Calories

BLOOD SUGAR LOG

	Blood Sugar Level	
	Before	**After**
WAKING UP Time: _____	Sleep Hrs: _____ Fast. Hrs: _____	
BREAKFAST		
SNACK 1		
LUNCH		
SNACK 2		
DINNER		
BEDTIME	Go to Sleep Time: _____	

BLOOD PRESSURE & WEIGHT

Time	SYS/DIA	Pulse

WEIGHT: _____

NOTES/SCHEDULE

7 am	
8 am	
9 am	
10 am	
11 am	
12 am	
1 pm	
2 pm	
3 pm	
4 pm	
5 pm	
6 pm	
7 pm	
8 pm	

DATE: _____ SU | MO | TU | WE | TH | FR | SA   **Month/Week:** _____

FOOD, NUTRITION & MEDS

	Carbs	Sugar	Fiber	Protein	Fat	Calories
BREAKFAST Time: _____ Meds/Insulin: _____						
Breakfast Total						
SNACK 1 Time: _____ Meds/Insulin: _____						
Snack 1 Total						
LUNCH Time: _____ Meds/Insulin: _____						
Lunch Total						
SNACK 2 Time: _____ Meds/Insulin: _____						
Snack 2 Total						
DINNER Time: _____ Meds/Insulin: _____						
Dinner Total						
Total Nutrition for the Day						

Water Consumption ▯▯▯▯▯▯▯▯▯▯ _____

EXERCISE & ACTIVITY LOG

	Time/Duration	Intensity/Calories

BLOOD SUGAR LOG

	Blood Sugar Level	
	Before	**After**
WAKING UP Time: _____	Sleep Hrs: _____ Fast. Hrs: _____	
BREAKFAST		
SNACK 1		
LUNCH		
SNACK 2		
DINNER		
BEDTIME	Go to Sleep Time: _____	

BLOOD PRESSURE & WEIGHT

Time	SYS/DIA	Pulse

WEIGHT: _____

NOTES/SCHEDULE

7 am	
8 am	
9 am	
10 am	
11 am	
12 am	
1 pm	
2 pm	
3 pm	
4 pm	
5 pm	
6 pm	
7 pm	
8 pm	

DATE: _____   SU | MO | TU | WE | TH | FR | SA   **Month/Week:** _____

FOOD, NUTRITION & MEDS

	Carbs	Sugar	Fiber	Protein	Fat	Calories

BREAKFAST   Time: _____   Meds/Insulin: _____

Breakfast Total						

SNACK 1   Time: _____   Meds/Insulin: _____

Snack 1 Total						

LUNCH   Time: _____   Meds/Insulin: _____

Lunch Total						

SNACK 2   Time: _____   Meds/Insulin: _____

Snack 2 Total						

DINNER   Time: _____   Meds/Insulin: _____

Dinner Total						
Total Nutrition for the Day						

Water Consumption ⬜⬜⬜⬜⬜⬜⬜⬜⬜⬜ _____

BLOOD SUGAR LOG

	Blood Sugar Level	
	Before	**After**
WAKING UP Time: _____	Sleep Hrs: _____ Fast. Hrs: _____	
BREAKFAST		
SNACK 1		
LUNCH		
SNACK 2		
DINNER		
BEDTIME	Go to Sleep Time: _____	

BLOOD PRESSURE & WEIGHT

Time	**SYS/DIA**	**Pulse**

WEIGHT: _____

NOTES/SCHEDULE

7 am	
8 am	
9 am	
10 am	
11 am	
12 am	
1 pm	
2 pm	
3 pm	
4 pm	
5 pm	
6 pm	
7 pm	
8 pm	

EXERCISE & ACTIVITY LOG

	Time/Duration	**Intensity/Calories**

DATE: _____   SU | MO | TU | WE | TH | FR | SA   **Month/Week:** _____

FOOD, NUTRITION & MEDS

	Carbs	Sugar	Fiber	Protein	Fat	Calories
BREAKFAST Time: _____ Meds/Insulin: _____						
Breakfast Total						
SNACK 1 Time: _____ Meds/Insulin: _____						
Snack 1 Total						
LUNCH Time: _____ Meds/Insulin: _____						
Lunch Total						
SNACK 2 Time: _____ Meds/Insulin: _____						
Snack 2 Total						
DINNER Time: _____ Meds/Insulin: _____						
Dinner Total						
Total Nutrition for the Day						

Water Consumption ⬜⬜⬜⬜⬜⬜⬜⬜⬜⬜ _____

EXERCISE & ACTIVITY LOG

	Time/Duration	Intensity/Calories

BLOOD SUGAR LOG

	Blood Sugar Level	
	Before	**After**
WAKING UP Time: _____	Sleep Hrs: _____ Fast. Hrs: _____	
BREAKFAST		
SNACK 1		
LUNCH		
SNACK 2		
DINNER		
BEDTIME	Go to Sleep Time: _____	

BLOOD PRESSURE & WEIGHT

Time	SYS/DIA	Pulse

WEIGHT: _____

NOTES/SCHEDULE

7 am	
8 am	
9 am	
10 am	
11 am	
12 am	
1 pm	
2 pm	
3 pm	
4 pm	
5 pm	
6 pm	
7 pm	
8 pm	

DATE: _____ SU | MO | TU | WE | TH | FR | SA   **Month/Week:** _____

FOOD, NUTRITION & MEDS

		Carbs	Sugar	Fiber	Protein	Fat	Calories
BREAKFAST Time: _____ Meds/Insulin: _____							
	Breakfast Total						
SNACK 1 Time: _____ Meds/Insulin: _____							
	Snack 1 Total						
LUNCH Time: _____ Meds/Insulin: _____							
	Lunch Total						
SNACK 2 Time: _____ Meds/Insulin: _____							
	Snack 2 Total						
DINNER Time: _____ Meds/Insulin: _____							
	Dinner Total						
	Total Nutrition for the Day						

Water Consumption ⬜⬜⬜⬜⬜⬜⬜⬜⬜ _____

BLOOD SUGAR LOG

	Blood Sugar Level	
	Before	**After**
WAKING UP Time: _____	Sleep Hrs: _____ Fast. Hrs: _____	
BREAKFAST		
SNACK 1		
LUNCH		
SNACK 2		
DINNER		
BEDTIME	Go to Sleep Time: _____	

BLOOD PRESSURE & WEIGHT

Time	SYS/DIA	Pulse

WEIGHT: _____

NOTES/SCHEDULE

7 am	
8 am	
9 am	
10 am	
11 am	
12 am	
1 pm	
2 pm	
3 pm	
4 pm	
5 pm	
6 pm	
7 pm	
8 pm	

EXERCISE & ACTIVITY LOG

	Time/Duration	Intensity/Calories

DATE: _____ SU | MO | TU | WE | TH | FR | SA

Month/Week: _____

FOOD, NUTRITION & MEDS

		Carbs	Sugar	Fiber	Protein	Fat	Calories
BREAKFAST Time: _____ Meds/Insulin: _____							
	Breakfast Total						
SNACK 1 Time: _____ Meds/Insulin: _____							
	Snack 1 Total						
LUNCH Time: _____ Meds/Insulin: _____							
	Lunch Total						
SNACK 2 Time: _____ Meds/Insulin: _____							
	Snack 2 Total						
DINNER Time: _____ Meds/Insulin: _____							
	Dinner Total						
	Total Nutrition for the Day						

Water Consumption ⬜⬜⬜⬜⬜⬜⬜⬜⬜ _____

EXERCISE & ACTIVITY LOG

	Time/Duration	Intensity/Calories

BLOOD SUGAR LOG

	Blood Sugar Level	
	Before	**After**
WAKING UP Time: _____	Sleep Hrs: _____ Fast. Hrs: _____	
BREAKFAST		
SNACK 1		
LUNCH		
SNACK 2		
DINNER		
BEDTIME	Go to Sleep Time: _____	

BLOOD PRESSURE & WEIGHT

Time	SYS/DIA	Pulse

WEIGHT: _____

NOTES/SCHEDULE

7 am	
8 am	
9 am	
10 am	
11 am	
12 am	
1 pm	
2 pm	
3 pm	
4 pm	
5 pm	
6 pm	
7 pm	
8 pm	

DATE: _____   SU | MO | TU | WE | TH | FR | SA   **Month/Week:** _____

FOOD, NUTRITION & MEDS

		Carbs	Sugar	Fiber	Protein	Fat	Calories
BREAKFAST Time: _____ Meds/Insulin: _____							
	Breakfast Total						
SNACK 1 Time: _____ Meds/Insulin: _____							
	Snack 1 Total						
LUNCH Time: _____ Meds/Insulin: _____							
	Lunch Total						
SNACK 2 Time: _____ Meds/Insulin: _____							
	Snack 2 Total						
DINNER Time: _____ Meds/Insulin: _____							
	Dinner Total						
	Total Nutrition for the Day						

Water Consumption ⊔ ⊔ ⊔ ⊔ ⊔ ⊔ ⊔ ⊔ ⊔   _____

BLOOD SUGAR LOG

	Blood Sugar Level	
	Before	**After**
WAKING UP Time: _____	Sleep Hrs: _____ Fast. Hrs: _____	
BREAKFAST		
SNACK 1		
LUNCH		
SNACK 2		
DINNER		
BEDTIME	Go to Sleep Time: _____	

BLOOD PRESSURE & WEIGHT

Time	SYS/DIA	Pulse
WEIGHT: _____		

NOTES/SCHEDULE

7 am	
8 am	
9 am	
10 am	
11 am	
12 am	
1 pm	
2 pm	
3 pm	
4 pm	
5 pm	
6 pm	
7 pm	
8 pm	

EXERCISE & ACTIVITY LOG

	Time/Duration	Intensity/Calories

DATE: _____ SU | MO | TU | WE | TH | FR | SA   **Month/Week:** _____

FOOD, NUTRITION & MEDS

	Carbs	Sugar	Fiber	Protein	Fat	Calories
BREAKFAST Time: _____ Meds/Insulin: _____						
Breakfast Total						
SNACK 1 Time: _____ Meds/Insulin: _____						
Snack 1 Total						
LUNCH Time: _____ Meds/Insulin: _____						
Lunch Total						
SNACK 2 Time: _____ Meds/Insulin: _____						
Snack 2 Total						
DINNER Time: _____ Meds/Insulin: _____						
Dinner Total						
Total Nutrition for the Day						

Water Consumption ⬜⬜⬜⬜⬜⬜⬜⬜⬜⬜ _____

EXERCISE & ACTIVITY LOG

	Time/Duration	Intensity/Calories

BLOOD SUGAR LOG

	Blood Sugar Level	
	Before	**After**
WAKING UP Time: _____	Sleep Hrs: _____ Fast. Hrs: _____	
BREAKFAST		
SNACK 1		
LUNCH		
SNACK 2		
DINNER		
BEDTIME	Go to Sleep Time: _____	

BLOOD PRESSURE & WEIGHT

Time	SYS/DIA	Pulse

WEIGHT: _____

NOTES/SCHEDULE

7 am	
8 am	
9 am	
10 am	
11 am	
12 am	
1 pm	
2 pm	
3 pm	
4 pm	
5 pm	
6 pm	
7 pm	
8 pm	

DATE: _____ SU | MO | TU | WE | TH | FR | SA   **Month/Week:** _____

FOOD, NUTRITION & MEDS

	Carbs	Sugar	Fiber	Protein	Fat	Calories
BREAKFAST Time: _____ Meds/Insulin: _____						
Breakfast Total						
SNACK 1 Time: _____ Meds/Insulin: _____						
Snack 1 Total						
LUNCH Time: _____ Meds/Insulin: _____						
Lunch Total						
SNACK 2 Time: _____ Meds/Insulin: _____						
Snack 2 Total						
DINNER Time: _____ Meds/Insulin: _____						
Dinner Total						
Total Nutrition for the Day						

Water Consumption ⬚ ⬚ ⬚ ⬚ ⬚ ⬚ ⬚ ⬚ ⬚ ⬚ _____

EXERCISE & ACTIVITY LOG

	Time/Duration	Intensity/Calories

BLOOD SUGAR LOG

	Blood Sugar Level	
	Before	**After**
WAKING UP Time: _____	Sleep Hrs: _____ Fast. Hrs: _____	
BREAKFAST		
SNACK 1		
LUNCH		
SNACK 2		
DINNER		
BEDTIME	Go to Sleep Time: _____	

BLOOD PRESSURE & WEIGHT

Time	SYS/DIA	Pulse

WEIGHT: _____

NOTES/SCHEDULE

7 am	
8 am	
9 am	
10 am	
11 am	
12 am	
1 pm	
2 pm	
3 pm	
4 pm	
5 pm	
6 pm	
7 pm	
8 pm	

DATE: _____ SU | MO | TU | WE | TH | FR | SA **Month/Week:** _____

FOOD, NUTRITION & MEDS

	Carbs	Sugar	Fiber	Protein	Fat	Calories
BREAKFAST Time: _____ Meds/Insulin: _____						
Breakfast Total						
SNACK 1 Time: _____ Meds/Insulin: _____						
Snack 1 Total						
LUNCH Time: _____ Meds/Insulin: _____						
Lunch Total						
SNACK 2 Time: _____ Meds/Insulin: _____						
Snack 2 Total						
DINNER Time: _____ Meds/Insulin: _____						
Dinner Total						
Total Nutrition for the Day						

Water Consumption 🥛🥛🥛🥛🥛🥛🥛🥛🥛 _____

BLOOD SUGAR LOG

	Blood Sugar Level	
	Before	**After**
WAKING UP Time: _____	Sleep Hrs: _____ Fast. Hrs: _____	
BREAKFAST		
SNACK 1		
LUNCH		
SNACK 2		
DINNER		
BEDTIME	Go to Sleep Time: _____	

BLOOD PRESSURE & WEIGHT

Time	SYS/DIA	Pulse

WEIGHT: _____

NOTES/SCHEDULE

7 am	
8 am	
9 am	
10 am	
11 am	
12 am	
1 pm	
2 pm	
3 pm	
4 pm	
5 pm	
6 pm	
7 pm	
8 pm	

EXERCISE & ACTIVITY LOG

	Time/Duration	Intensity/Calories

DATE: _____   SU | MO | TU | WE | TH | FR | SA   **Month/Week:** _____

FOOD, NUTRITION & MEDS

		Carbs	Sugar	Fiber	Protein	Fat	Calories
BREAKFAST Time: _____ Meds/Insulin: _____							
	Breakfast Total						
SNACK 1 Time: _____ Meds/Insulin: _____							
	Snack 1 Total						
LUNCH Time: _____ Meds/Insulin: _____							
	Lunch Total						
SNACK 2 Time: _____ Meds/Insulin: _____							
	Snack 2 Total						
DINNER Time: _____ Meds/Insulin: _____							
	Dinner Total						
	Total Nutrition for the Day						

Water Consumption ⬜ ⬜ ⬜ ⬜ ⬜ ⬜ ⬜ ⬜ ⬜ _____

BLOOD SUGAR LOG

		Blood Sugar Level	
		Before	**After**
WAKING UP Time: _____	Sleep Hrs: _____ Fast. Hrs: _____		
BREAKFAST			
SNACK 1			
LUNCH			
SNACK 2			
DINNER			
BEDTIME	Go to Sleep Time: _____		

BLOOD PRESSURE & WEIGHT

Time	SYS/DIA	Pulse

WEIGHT: _____

NOTES/SCHEDULE

7 am	
8 am	
9 am	
10 am	
11 am	
12 am	
1 pm	
2 pm	
3 pm	
4 pm	
5 pm	
6 pm	
7 pm	
8 pm	

EXERCISE & ACTIVITY LOG

	Time/Duration	Intensity/Calories

DATE: _ _ _ _ _ _ _ _ _ _ _ _ _ _ _ _ _   SU | MO | TU | WE | TH | FR | SA   **Month/Week:** _ _ _ _ _ _ _ _ _ _ _ _ _ _ _ _ _

FOOD, NUTRITION & MEDS

	Carbs	Sugar	Fiber	Protein	Fat	Calories
BREAKFAST Time: _ _ _ _ _ _ _ _ _ Meds/Insulin: _						
Breakfast Total						
SNACK 1 Time: _ _ _ _ _ _ _ _ _ Meds/Insulin: _ _ _ _ _ _ _ _ _ _ _ _ _ _ _ _ _ _						
Snack 1 Total						
LUNCH Time: _ _ _ _ _ _ _ _ _ Meds/Insulin: _ _ _ _ _ _ _ _ _ _ _ _ _ _ _ _ _ _						
Lunch Total						
SNACK 2 Time: _ _ _ _ _ _ _ _ _ Meds/Insulin: _ _ _ _ _ _ _ _ _ _ _ _ _ _ _ _ _ _						
Snack 2 Total						
DINNER Time: _ _ _ _ _ _ _ _ _ Meds/Insulin: _ _ _ _ _ _ _ _ _ _ _ _ _ _ _ _ _ _						
Dinner Total						
Total Nutrition for the Day						

Water Consumption ☐ ☐ ☐ ☐ ☐ ☐ ☐ ☐ ☐ ☐ _ _ _ _ _ _ _ _ _ _ _ _ _

EXERCISE & ACTIVITY LOG

	Time/Duration	Intensity/Calories

BLOOD SUGAR LOG

	Blood Sugar Level	
	Before	**After**
WAKING UP Time: _ _ _ _ _ _ _	Sleep Hrs: _ _ _ _ _ _ _ _ _ _ _ Fast. Hrs: _ _ _ _ _ _ _ _ _ _ _	
BREAKFAST		
SNACK 1		
LUNCH		
SNACK 2		
DINNER		
BEDTIME	Go to Sleep Time: _ _ _ _ _ _ _ _ _ _ _	

BLOOD PRESSURE & WEIGHT

Time	SYS/DIA	Pulse

WEIGHT: _

NOTES/SCHEDULE

7 am	
8 am	
9 am	
10 am	
11 am	
12 am	
1 pm	
2 pm	
3 pm	
4 pm	
5 pm	
6 pm	
7 pm	
8 pm	

DATE: _____ SU | MO | TU | WE | TH | FR | SA   **Month/Week:** _____

FOOD, NUTRITION & MEDS

		Carbs	Sugar	Fiber	Protein	Fat	Calories
BREAKFAST Time: _____	Meds/Insulin: _____						
	Breakfast Total						
SNACK 1 Time: _____	Meds/Insulin: _____						
	Snack 1 Total						
LUNCH Time: _____	Meds/Insulin: _____						
	Lunch Total						
SNACK 2 Time: _____	Meds/Insulin: _____						
	Snack 2 Total						
DINNER Time: _____	Meds/Insulin: _____						
	Dinner Total						
	Total Nutrition for the Day						

Water Consumption ▭ ▭ ▭ ▭ ▭ ▭ ▭ ▭ ▭   _____

BLOOD SUGAR LOG

	Blood Sugar Level	
	Before	**After**
WAKING UP Time: _____	Sleep Hrs: _____ Fast. Hrs: _____	
BREAKFAST		
SNACK 1		
LUNCH		
SNACK 2		
DINNER		
BEDTIME	Go to Sleep Time: _____	

BLOOD PRESSURE & WEIGHT

Time	**SYS/DIA**	**Pulse**

WEIGHT: _____

NOTES/SCHEDULE

7 am	
8 am	
9 am	
10 am	
11 am	
12 am	
1 pm	
2 pm	
3 pm	
4 pm	
5 pm	
6 pm	
7 pm	
8 pm	

EXERCISE & ACTIVITY LOG

	Time/Duration	**Intensity/Calories**

DATE: _____ SU | MO | TU | WE | TH | FR | SA

Month/Week: _____

FOOD, NUTRITION & MEDS

	Carbs	Sugar	Fiber	Protein	Fat	Calories
BREAKFAST Time: _____ Meds/Insulin: _____						
Breakfast Total						
SNACK 1 Time: _____ Meds/Insulin: _____						
Snack 1 Total						
LUNCH Time: _____ Meds/Insulin: _____						
Lunch Total						
SNACK 2 Time: _____ Meds/Insulin: _____						
Snack 2 Total						
DINNER Time: _____ Meds/Insulin: _____						
Dinner Total						
Total Nutrition for the Day						

Water Consumption ⊔ ⊔ ⊔ ⊔ ⊔ ⊔ ⊔ ⊔ ⊔ ⊔ _____

EXERCISE & ACTIVITY LOG

	Time/Duration	Intensity/Calories

BLOOD SUGAR LOG

	Blood Sugar Level	
	Before	After
WAKING UP Time: _____	Sleep Hrs: _____ Fast. Hrs: _____	
BREAKFAST		
SNACK 1		
LUNCH		
SNACK 2		
DINNER		
BEDTIME	Go to Sleep Time: _____	

BLOOD PRESSURE & WEIGHT

Time	SYS/DIA	Pulse

WEIGHT: _____

NOTES/SCHEDULE

7 am	
8 am	
9 am	
10 am	
11 am	
12 am	
1 pm	
2 pm	
3 pm	
4 pm	
5 pm	
6 pm	
7 pm	
8 pm	

DATE: _____   SU | MO | TU | WE | TH | FR | SA   **Month/Week:** _____

FOOD, NUTRITION & MEDS

	Carbs	Sugar	Fiber	Protein	Fat	Calories
BREAKFAST Time: _____ Meds/Insulin: _____						
Breakfast Total						
SNACK 1 Time: _____ Meds/Insulin: _____						
Snack 1 Total						
LUNCH Time: _____ Meds/Insulin: _____						
Lunch Total						
SNACK 2 Time: _____ Meds/Insulin: _____						
Snack 2 Total						
DINNER Time: _____ Meds/Insulin: _____						
Dinner Total						
Total Nutrition for the Day						

Water Consumption ▢ ▢ ▢ ▢ ▢ ▢ ▢ ▢ ▢ ▢ _____

EXERCISE & ACTIVITY LOG

	Time/Duration	Intensity/Calories

BLOOD SUGAR LOG

	Blood Sugar Level	
	Before	**After**
WAKING UP Time: _____	Sleep Hrs: _____ Fast. Hrs: _____	
BREAKFAST		
SNACK 1		
LUNCH		
SNACK 2		
DINNER		
BEDTIME	Go to Sleep Time: _____	

BLOOD PRESSURE & WEIGHT

Time	SYS/DIA	Pulse
WEIGHT: _____		

NOTES/SCHEDULE

7 am	
8 am	
9 am	
10 am	
11 am	
12 am	
1 pm	
2 pm	
3 pm	
4 pm	
5 pm	
6 pm	
7 pm	
8 pm	

DATE: _ _ _ _ _ _ _ _ _ _ _ _ _ _ _ _ SU | MO | TU | WE | TH | FR | SA

Month/Week: _ _ _ _ _ _ _ _ _ _ _ _ _ _ _ _

FOOD, NUTRITION & MEDS

	Carbs	Sugar	Fiber	Protein	Fat	Calories
BREAKFAST Time: _ _ _ _ _ _ Meds/Insulin: _ _ _ _ _ _ _ _ _ _ _						
Breakfast Total						
SNACK 1 Time: _ _ _ _ _ _ Meds/Insulin: _ _ _ _ _ _ _ _ _ _ _						
Snack 1 Total						
LUNCH Time: _ _ _ _ _ _ Meds/Insulin: _ _ _ _ _ _ _ _ _ _ _						
Lunch Total						
SNACK 2 Time: _ _ _ _ _ _ Meds/Insulin: _ _ _ _ _ _ _ _ _ _ _						
Snack 2 Total						
DINNER Time: _ _ _ _ _ _ Meds/Insulin: _ _ _ _ _ _ _ _ _ _ _						
Dinner Total						
Total Nutrition for the Day						

Water Consumption ⬜⬜⬜⬜⬜⬜⬜⬜⬜⬜ _ _ _ _ _ _ _

BLOOD SUGAR LOG

	Blood Sugar Level	
	Before	**After**
WAKING UP Time: _ _ _ _ _	Sleep Hrs: _ _ _ _ _ Fast. Hrs: _ _ _ _ _	
BREAKFAST		
SNACK 1		
LUNCH		
SNACK 2		
DINNER		
BEDTIME	Go to Sleep Time: _ _ _ _ _	

BLOOD PRESSURE & WEIGHT

Time	SYS/DIA	Pulse
WEIGHT: _ _ _ _ _ _ _ _		

NOTES/SCHEDULE

7 am	
8 am	
9 am	
10 am	
11 am	
12 am	
1 pm	
2 pm	
3 pm	
4 pm	
5 pm	
6 pm	
7 pm	
8 pm	

EXERCISE & ACTIVITY LOG

	Time/Duration	Intensity/Calories

DATE: _____ SU | MO | TU | WE | TH | FR | SA   **Month/Week:** _____

FOOD, NUTRITION & MEDS

	Carbs	Sugar	Fiber	Protein	Fat	Calories
BREAKFAST Time: _____ Meds/Insulin: _____						
Breakfast Total						
SNACK 1 Time: _____ Meds/Insulin: _____						
Snack 1 Total						
LUNCH Time: _____ Meds/Insulin: _____						
Lunch Total						
SNACK 2 Time: _____ Meds/Insulin: _____						
Snack 2 Total						
DINNER Time: _____ Meds/Insulin: _____						
Dinner Total						
Total Nutrition for the Day						

Water Consumption ▯ ▯ ▯ ▯ ▯ ▯ ▯ ▯ ▯ ▯ _____

BLOOD SUGAR LOG

	Blood Sugar Level	
	Before	**After**
WAKING UP Time: _____	Sleep Hrs: _____ Fast. Hrs: _____	
BREAKFAST		
SNACK 1		
LUNCH		
SNACK 2		
DINNER		
BEDTIME	Go to Sleep Time: _____	

BLOOD PRESSURE & WEIGHT

Time	SYS/DIA	Pulse

WEIGHT: _____

NOTES/SCHEDULE

7 am	
8 am	
9 am	
10 am	
11 am	
12 am	
1 pm	
2 pm	
3 pm	
4 pm	
5 pm	
6 pm	
7 pm	
8 pm	

EXERCISE & ACTIVITY LOG

	Time/Duration	Intensity/Calories

DATE: _____ SU | MO | TU | WE | TH | FR | SA

Month/Week: _____

FOOD, NUTRITION & MEDS

	Carbs	Sugar	Fiber	Protein	Fat	Calories
BREAKFAST Time: _____ Meds/Insulin: _____						
Breakfast Total						
SNACK 1 Time: _____ Meds/Insulin: _____						
Snack 1 Total						
LUNCH Time: _____ Meds/Insulin: _____						
Lunch Total						
SNACK 2 Time: _____ Meds/Insulin: _____						
Snack 2 Total						
DINNER Time: _____ Meds/Insulin: _____						
Dinner Total						
Total Nutrition for the Day						

Water Consumption ⊔ ⊔ ⊔ ⊔ ⊔ ⊔ ⊔ ⊔ ⊔ ⊔   _____

EXERCISE & ACTIVITY LOG

	Time/Duration	Intensity/Calories

BLOOD SUGAR LOG

	Blood Sugar Level	
	Before	**After**
WAKING UP Time: _____	Sleep Hrs: _____ Fast. Hrs: _____	
BREAKFAST		
SNACK 1		
LUNCH		
SNACK 2		
DINNER		
BEDTIME	Go to Sleep Time: _____	

BLOOD PRESSURE & WEIGHT

Time	SYS/DIA	Pulse

WEIGHT: _____

NOTES/SCHEDULE

7 am	
8 am	
9 am	
10 am	
11 am	
12 am	
1 pm	
2 pm	
3 pm	
4 pm	
5 pm	
6 pm	
7 pm	
8 pm	

Medical Notes

Medical Notes

Medical Notes

Medical Notes

Made in the USA
Las Vegas, NV
25 October 2023